PRIMITIVE PHYSIC

by

JOHN WESLEY

with an

INTRODUCTION

by

A. WESLEY HILL

LONDON
THE EPWORTH PRESS

FIRST PUBLISHED IN 1747
AND REPRINTED MANY TIMES
THIS EDITION PUBLISHED IN 1960

© THE EPWORTH PRESS 1960

Book Steward

FRANK H. CUMBERS

Printed and bound in England by Hazell Watson & Viney Ltd
Aylesbury and Slough

INTRODUCTION
by A. WESLEY HILL

JOHN WESLEY'S *Primitive Physic*, with its rules for good health and cures for various illnesses, was published and circulated in many editions, and played its part in meeting a need that challenged Wesley in his reforming work in the eighteenth century. He perceived and earnestly desired that his followers should have healthy bodies and healthy minds as well as saved souls. He therefore made sure that the humblest had access to wholesome literature for the cultivation of their minds, while, for the care of their bodies in sickness and in health, he provided in such a book as *Primitive Physic* an easy method of curing most diseases, and a guide to those 'who desire, through the blessing of God, to retain the health which they have recovered'.

Wesley and the Regular Physicians

Why did he not leave this work of attending to the sick and ailing to the regular physicians of that day? Why must he undertake what others were better trained and qualified to do? A good part of the answer to this question is found in his Preface to *Primitive Physic*. Before dealing with that Preface however, we must remind ourselves that he was himself well qualified, both in disposition and in knowledge, for this work. There were few better qualified. This is not so surprising when we realize that eighteenth-century medical knowledge in its entirety was well within the compass of any gentleman's ordinary education. Richard Baxter (1615–91) was not only parish minister of Kidderminster but also a successful medical practitioner. J. H. Whiteley[1] lists many reverend gentlemen who were physicians of the body as well as of the soul. Crabbe was poet, clergyman and doctor; Horne Tooke studied medicine for the benefit of his poor parishioners; the Reverend Doctor Stukley was physician as well as vicar; Rowland Hill had an

---

[1] *Wesley's Anglican Contemporaries*, pp. 37–8.

3

enthusiasm for innoculation; and Bishop Berkeley, philanthropist and philosopher, made Tar Water one of the most popular of eighteenth-century remedies. Indeed for the most part the poor folk in country districts had no one to look to in their sicknesses but the squire or vicar, and, more often than not, had to be content with their own local traditional simples. Even when a regular physician was available they were not likely to be able to pay his fee.

Wesley was an ardent reader of the medical literature of his day. 'For six or seven and twenty years I had made Anatomy and Physic the diversion of my leisure hours: though I never properly studied them, unless for a few months when I was going to America, where I imagined I might be of some service to those who had no regular physician among them. I applied to it again.'[1] This reading, applied in practice to the treatment of illness both at the dispensaries he opened and during his travels, made him expert both in diagnosis and treatment. There is ample evidence that he was quite capable of undertaking the office of physician.

Beyond all this, however, was Wesley's distrust both of the physicians and the hospitals of his day, a distrust which is seen very clearly in his Preface to *Primitive Physic*, which contains a serious indictment of most of the contemporary medical profession. This Preface is an integral part of *Primitive Physic*, and to publish the remedies or any selection of them without it would be to wrong Wesley. Samples of the best type of eighteenth-century remedies as they are, they have little or no therapeutic value today, and would by themselves expose Wesley, their editor, to the condescending smile that properly belongs to extracts from eighteenth-century pharmacopoeias; but the Preface together with this collection of remedies throws important light on eighteenth-century medicine and the part Wesley played in it. Lack of study and understanding of this Preface has led many not only to misinterpret the title *Primitive Physic*, but also to underestimate the necessary and the pioneering work of Wesley in his role of physician. An attempt, therefore, to expound the Preface and to give some account of

[1] *Letters of John Wesley* (Standard Edition), II. 307.

4

the philosophies against which it inveighs will now be entered upon.

The Origin of Disease

Wesley accepted the Genesis story of Creation as historical and as having happened within measurable time. His thought was not troubled by the idea of medicine's slow climb upwards through animistic taboos and exorcisms. He was a man of his age. His contemporary Dr John Brown in his *Elementa Medicinae* could aptly reinforce an argument by reference to Holy Writ: '*Hinc primae hominis maledictionis facilis explicatio, Quo die comederis eo profecto morieris.*'[1] We are, therefore, not surprised when Wesley begins his Preface with a description of a perfection of creation so soon marred by

> *Man's first disobedience and the fruit*
> *Of that forbidden tree, whose mortal taste*
> *Brought death into the world and all our woe.*

For Wesley, 'When man came first out of the hands of the great Creator, . . . there was no place for physic, or the art of healing. As he knew no sin, so he knew no pain, no sickness, weakness, or bodily disorder. . . . well might *the morning-stars sing together, and all the sons of* God *shout for joy.*' Wesley saw man as normally perfect, and, though marred by sin in body, mind and soul, as capable of being restored to that original perfection. He did not look at disease as an entity in itself; he saw diseased man as a departure from the normal, since his body originally 'had no seeds of corruption or dissolution within itself. And there was nothing without to injure it.'

From this point Wesley paints the picture of the results of man's fall from divine favour. 'The heavens, the earth, and all things contained therein, conspire to punish the rebels against their Creator. The sun and moon shed unwholesome influences from above; the earth exhales poisonous damps from beneath: . . . the air itself that surrounds us on every side, is replete with the shafts of death.' He sees here a conspiracy of

[1] From this arises an easy interpretation of that primal curse upon mankind—In the day thou eatest therefore thou shalt surely die.

5

nature against man—sunstroke and lunacy descending from above, paludal mal-aria lifting from below, and an environment loaded with lethal micro-organisms.

The Discovery of Cures

Wesley believed in the mercy as well as the justice of the Creator. Apart from that belief he would have had no evangel either for the body or the soul. With St Paul he believed that God always will with the trial make also the way of escape, and that alongside the poison there will be found an antidote. So he confidently inquires, 'Can nothing be found to lessen these inconveniences which cannot be wholly removed?' and he promptly discovers a prophylactic blessing wrapped up in the divine malediction itself: ' "In the sweat of thy face shalt thou eat bread, till thou return to the ground." The power of exercise, both to preserve and restore health, is greater than can well be conceived.'

Here Wesley secures for himself a scriptural basis for his thesis that cures can and should be discovered by accident and proved by experience, and that this is the way the healing art grows. He sees this in what he regards as the beginning of human history. This way of discovering cures and experimenting with them was the primitive way by which was gathered up the whole corpus of healing. 'It is probable Physic as well as Religion was in the first ages chiefly traditional, every father delivering down to his sons what he had in like manner received concerning the manner of healing both inward hurts and the diseases incident to each climate, and the medicines which were of the greatest efficacy for the cure of each disorder.' This is what Wesley means by 'Primitive Physic'.

This conception of primitive physic has been reinforced by observation of the customs of North American Indians whom he has met during his residence in Georgia. Here he has been observing at first hand a primitive race, and he sees that 'this is the method wherein the art of healing is preserved among the *Americans* to this day. Their diseases indeed are exceeding few; nor do they often occur by reason of their continual exercise, and (till of late) universal temperance. But if any are

6

sick, or bit by a serpent, or torn by a wild beast, the fathers immediately tell their children what remedy to apply. And it is rare, that the patient suffers long; those medicines being quick, as well as generally infallible.'

It is this simple procedure of discovery of cure, experience of its utility or inutility, and the handing on through the generations of what proves to be effective, which Wesley opposes to the fantastic hypotheses which, from the time of the speculative Greeks until after the close of the eighteenth century, formed accepted explanations of health and disease, and dominated methods of treatment. Interesting as ingenious speculations and as attempts to fill the gap of ignorance about true causes of disease, these hypotheses were yet fatal to the true advancement of medical knowledge and the discovery of effective medical treatment. If a true knowledge of what causes a disease—for example, the knowledge that measles is caused by a virus—does not necessarily suggest a cure, how much less can erroneous philosophies dictate one? It was not indeed until these outworn theories of disease were finally discarded in the early nineteenth century, and what Wesley called the method of primitive physic was resumed, that the modern age of medical progress dawned.

Here is how Wesley sets the matter forth. 'Thus far physic was wholly founded on experiment. The *European*, as well as the *American* [Indian], said to his neighbour, Are you sick? Drink the juice of this herb, and your sickness will be at an end. . . . Thus ancient men, having a little experience joined with common sense, and common humanity, cured both themselves and their neighbours of most of the distempers, to which every nation was subject.'

This experimental, traditional way has always been the way of medical progress. Centuries ago Colchicum was found to be a cure for gout. A little while ago Phenylbutazone was discovered also to be a cure for gout—though the mode of action of neither of these drugs in this disease is known. Specific cures, such as the antibiotic moulds, are still come upon by accident, as they were in ancient days, by those who are alert for such discovery. 'Has not the Author of Nature,' says our Preface, 'taught us the use of many other medicines, by what is vulgarly termed Accident?'

Criticism of the Medical Profession

'But in process of time,' continues Wesley, 'men of a philosophical turn were not satisfied with this. They began to enquire how they might *account* for these things? How such Medicines wrought such effects? . . . Men of learning began to set experience aside; to build physic upon hypothesis; to form theories of diseases and their cure, and to substitute these in the place of experiments.

'As theories increased, simple medicines were more and more disregarded and disused: till in a course of years, the greater part of them were forgotten, at least in the politer nations. In the room of these, abundance of new ones were introduced by reasoning, speculative men: and those more and more difficult to be applied, as being more remote from common observation. Hence rules for the application of these, and medical books were immensely multiplied; till at length physic became an abstruse science, quite out of reach of ordinary men.'

Before outlining some of the philosophies which Wesley had in mind, it must be noted that at this point the Preface goes on to make a sharper criticism. The medical profession is charged with deliberately adding to those difficulties of medical practice that had thus been built up, in order to increase its monopoly and its profit. 'To this end, they increased those difficulties by design, which began in a manner by accident. They filled their writings with abundance of technical terms, utterly unintelligible to plain men. They affected to deliver their rules, and to reason upon them, in an abstruse and philosophical manner. . . . They introduced into practice abundance of compound medicines, consisting of so many ingredients, that it was scarce possible for common people to know which it was that wrought the cure:[1] . . . yea, and of dangerous ones, such as they could not use without hazarding life, but by the advice of a physician. And thus

[1] A mixture regarded as effective against poisonous bites and known as Theriaca contained 60 to 70 substances pulverized and mixed with honey. An extreme example makes a good illustration.

8

both their honour and gain were secured, a vast majority of mankind being utterly cut off from helping either themselves or their neighbours, or once daring to attempt it.'

Wesley freely admits that all the profession was not thus guilty. 'There have not been wanting, from time to time, some lovers of mankind, who have endeavoured (even contrary to their own interest) to reduce physic to its ancient standard: who have laboured to explode it out of all the hypotheses and fine spun theories, and to make it a plain intelligible thing, as it was in the beginning: having no more mystery in it than this, "Such a medicine removes such a pain".' As examples of these 'lovers of mankind' he singles out such men as Sydenham, Dover, Cheyne, and Boerha[a]ve, but of the majority of physicians he speaks in irony as men who 'now began to be had in admiration, as persons who were something more than human'.

Eighteenth-century Theories about Disease

Let us now look first at some of the rules of medicine and then at some of the hypotheses of disease which Wesley deemed senseless and calculated to obstruct the natural accumulation of true therapeutic knowledge.

Lord Cohen in his Presidential Address before the Royal Society of Medicine[1] (26th October 1953) enumerated the four following doctrines about medicine—The Doctrine of Similars, The Doctrine of Signatures, The Doctrine of Analogy, and The Doctrine of Contagion.

The Doctrine of Similars would indicate that yellow birds, properly reduced to a medicament, were curative for jaundice, or that stewed raven prevented black hair from turning grey. This doctrine is not to be confused with the idea which forms the basis of homeopathy, namely, that a disease is best treated by administration of small quantities of those remedies which produce effects or symptoms similar to those produced by the disease itself. Hahnemann (1755–1843) was the founder of homeopathy and its method was expressed by the phrase *similia similibus curantur* ('Likes are cured by likes'). The Doctrine of Similars is to be distinguished from this.

[1] *The Evolution of the Concept of Disease.*

Paracelsus, a Swiss physician (1493–1541) whose real name was Theophrastus Bombastus, and Nicolas Culpeper are names associated with the Doctrine of Signatures, which teaches that medicines are best composed from those plants or animals whose markings suggest the part to be treated. Cyclamen, having the shape or signature of an ear, should be employed in treating an ear. Similarly, the liver-like shape of the leaf of liver-wort points to its use in hepatic disease. And again, the *New London Dispensatory* of 1682 tells us that the herb Euphrasia or Eyebright 'astringeth, discusseth, is sharp in taste and cephalic: the juyce or essence, both inwardly and outwardly used is good against Clouds, Mists, Pearls, Suffusions of the Eye and Loss of Memory'.

The Doctrine of Analogy was the most sensible of these rules, since it deduced cures from the behaviour of ailing animals. Wesley saw in it an excellent example of primitive physic. Agreeing with the Ancients that physic had a 'divine original', he says, 'It was a natural thought, That He who had taught it to the very beasts and birds, the *Cretan* Stag, the *Egyptian* Ibis, could not be wanting to teach man,

> *Sanctius his Animal, mentisque capacius altae:*[1]

Yea, sometimes by those meaner creatures: for it was easy to infer, 'If these will heal that creature, whose flesh is nearly of the same texture with mine, then in a parallel case it will heal me.'

On the other hand the Doctrine of Contagion is the most senseless. It found cures in things imagined to be associated with the cause of the distemper. A not inappropriate example of this teaching is that it recommended moonstone in the treatment of lunacy.

In the second place let us look at some of the Theories of Disease—those fantastic theories which 'men of a philosophical turn' introduced and which so seriously occupied the minds of medical men through centuries.

Take first the theory of the Methodist School. In the fourth century B.C. that remarkable philosopher Democritus

[1] Ovid, *Metamorphoses*, Bk. I, line 76: 'A being of more worth than these and more capable of lofty thought.'

taught that all matter is composed of indivisible particles, or atoms, and that all distinctions in matter arise from differences in the arrangement of these particles. Even the soul, he taught, is composed of atoms, albeit of finer and more subtle quality. This interesting and clever speculation became incorporated into medical history when Asclepiades (128–50 B.C.), a physician practising in Rome, developed from it an explanation of health and disease. When the body atoms are too widely spaced apart there results one kind of distemper; when they are too close together there follows another. This concept of disease was taken up by Themison of Laodicaea (c. 50 B.C.), who was the real founder of the School of Medicine known as the Methodist School. Fixing his attention on the pores or inter-atomic spaces, he too divided disease into two varieties. When the pores were of correct calibre and direction, so that body fluids could pass through them easily and properly, then a state of good health existed. But when the pores were constricted and distorted there followed that class of disease he called '*morbus strictus*', and when the pores were too open there resulted that class of disease he called '*morbus laxus*'.

With this hypothesis there was not only a neat division of disease into two classes, but the whole problem of cure became simple. Simplicity indeed was the motto of the Methodists. In the *strictus* class of disease one should employ relaxing agencies such as warmth, fomentations, laxatives, and very occasionally blood letting; in the *laxus* class one should employ astringents such as cold, alum, vinegar. Thus the whole business of therapy fell easily within the saying: '*Contraria Contrariis Curantur.*'

Here surely was the answer to the age-long desire of the human mind for an all-embracing formula that gathers within itself all the issues of life and death. Here was the philosopher's stone that turned the problem of health and disease into the shining gold of a great simplicity.

In actual practice the Methodists found that illnesses did not always readily fall into one or other of these groups, and the act of deciding to which one a disease belonged replaced automatic certainty by human fallibility. The inflamed eye with its con-stricted lid and copious tears must have presented what might

be described as a sticky problem for such choice.   In the end
many distempers had to be placed in an ever-growing mixed bag;
and symptoms, whether of *strictus* or *laxus* type, treated in the
order of urgency.   There grew up, however, a general agree-
ment, and diseases like asthma and epilepsy and melancholia
were regarded as *strictus*.   Caelius and Soranus, two noted
Methodists, decided that all cardiac diseases belonged to the *laxus*
variety, and consigned hydropsy and pleurisy and pneumonia to
the mixed class.

With varying fortune this School persisted until its last revival
in the eighteenth century, when Dr John Brown (1735–88)
published his *Elementa Medicinae*, the second edition of which,
with 'many emendations' was published in Edinburgh in 1784.
It is probable, from the entries in his diary, that this work en-
gaged the attention of John Wesley on the 6th and 7th Sep-
tember 1787.[1]

The second theory to be mentioned is the Brunonian one.
Dr John Brown, also, divided all diseases into two groups and
sought after simplicity in the classification of diseases and their
treatment.

He tells us that for more than twenty years he had been in-
vestigating medicine in all its aspects with great diligence.   He
divides his survey into four periods of five years each.   The
third lustrum found him 'in doubt and grief that nothing had
yet presented itself to his mind, and together with many eminent
men and the public itself, he lamented the health-giving art as
thoroughly unreliable and incomprehensible'. Only in the fourth
period of five years there dawned 'a dim light like that of earliest
day, as if upon a traveller in an unknown region who had lost all
traces of the road and was wandering amid the shades of night'.

The upshot of these painful and laborious cogitations was that
he saw diseases divided into two groups.   *'Communes omnes
morbus in duas formas, phlogisticam seu sthenicam et asthenicam
seu anti phlogisticam distribuit.'*[2]   The diseases he designates
sthenic arise from too much vigour; those he styles asthenic

[1] *The Journal of John Wesley* (Standard Edition), VII. 324.
[2] He divided all general diseases into two classes—inflammatory or sthenic
and anti-inflammatory or asthenic.

grow out of weakness. He finds, moreover, that many diseases formerly and by others regarded as due to excessive vigour in reality arise out of weakness.

As an example of this mistaken identity of origin he instances his own gout, which has been a starting-point for his investigations and which he now discovers belongs to the asthenic group. According to earlier opinion this disease sprang from plethora and excessive activity, and for its prevention wine was forbidden and a vegetable diet prescribed. His first attack came when he was thirty-six years of age and at a time when he had been on a meagre diet for a few months. Why had it not come in the years when he was living liberally and well? During this year of affliction with gout he lived on the low diet prescribed and had four most violent, painful and lengthy attacks of the disease. At length he made trial of the truth. Calling his friends together to breakfast, he drank merrily (*bibit hilariter*), 'and inside two hours had regained the full use of that foot with which before breakfast he had been unable to touch the floor for pain'.

Some diseases gave him difficulty in their allocation, and having at first put them in the sthenic group, he had them removed to the asthenic group in this second emended edition. In all this he knew that many of his findings were against accepted medical opinion, but he was convinced that the great Sydenham, although he had done so much to promote the treatment of inflammatory diseases (*phlogisticorum morborum*), was ignorant of asthenic diseases, 'having been led astray by alexipharmic[1] doctors' (*ab alexipharmacis medicis seductum*).

In the end Brown completed his lists of sthenic and asthenic diseases, and was quite satisfied that he had set forth a principle: '*Quod omnes partes illustrant et confirmant.*'[2] Like all the other philosophers about disease he considered that he had solved an age-long riddle, and by the art of inference (*ars conjecturalis*) had presented to the world something that 'might be called a science of life'.

Seen from the vantage ground of the twentieth century this is all great fun, but in those days these were important interests

[1] *Alexō*, to ward off + *pharmakon*, poison.
[2] Which every part illustrates and confirms.

and grave issues that were being raised. A sidelight on the seriousness with which the Brunonian theory was regarded was the quarrel between Dr William Cullen and its author that followed its publication. Brown had been Cullen's protégé, and owed nearly everything to him in his advance to the top ranks of his profession: between the two the most cordial friendship had existed. But now this book, with its division of disease into the sthenic and asthenic, had appeared at the moment when William Cullen was about to present to the world a classification of disease after the Linnaean pattern into classes, orders, genera and species.

Another set of theories may be called the Iatro group.[1] The Iatro-chemical theory held that all the phenomena of life were based on chemical action. The Iatro-physical or Iatro-mathematical held that all the phenomena of life were based on the laws of physics. This seemed specially designed to explain the circulation of the blood. Archibald Pitcairne (1652–1713), theologian, lawyer, mathematician, fellow of the Royal College of Physicians of Edinburgh at the age of twenty-seven, made such a name for himself as protagonist of this theory that he was invited to the Chair of Medicine of the famous Leyden University, where he numbered Boerhaave among his pupils.

A further hypothesis was the Pneumatic Theory. This was one of the more fantastic imaginings of 'men of a philosophical turn'. Athenaeus of Attalia, practising in Rome about the middle of the first century, taught that the pneuma or vital air was drawn into the lungs in breathing. This vital principle passed into the heart and arteries and was thus spread throughout the body. Its pulsation could be felt in the more superficial arteries and formed an indication of strength or weakness. Finally this vital principle was exhaled in death.

This theory persisted in many quarters long after Harvey had published his thesis on the circulation of the blood in 1628. It was hotly contested even after Marcello Malpighi in 1661 had demonstrated with his microscope the capillary beds connecting arteries and veins, thus finally establishing the fact of a closed system in which the blood could circulate.

[1] *Iatros*, physician.

Time would fail to describe in detail all the theories about health and disease that abounded in the eighteenth century, but there is one more which cannot be omitted if only because it was the most popular of them all. This is the Humoral Theory. It comes hoary with antiquity from Alkmaeon, the Pythagorean of Croton. It has the blessing of Hippocrates—though he was too wise to allow it seriously to influence his view of a particular disease or his method of expectant treatment. It was propagated by Galen. It is written into our language in such words as ill-humoured, sanguine, phlegmatic, jaundiced, melancholic (black bile). Some of us still remember the spring-time sulphur and treacle for purifying the blood.

The four elements of fire and earth and air and water matched the four qualities of heat and cold and dryness and moisture. With these a further correspondence was found in what were known as the four humours of the body—blood and phlegm and yellow bile and black bile. A right mixture or proportion of these humours constituted health; a wrong mixture or a wrong distribution of these constituted disease. The cold and dampness of winter cause an over-secretion in the brain of cold moist phlegm, which, falling down to the throat and lungs, causes laryngitis, bronchitis and pneumonia. The warm sunshine of spring causes the warm moist blood to mount to an excess. Always the cause of a disease could be traced, with semblance of solemn thought, to some redundancy of a humour. Hence arose treatment by purgings, vomits, and bleedings. The tragedy was that these notions about humours were so real and weighed so heavily on the minds and hearts of medical practitioners that this kind of treatment was often carried to an unreasonable extent and degree, even in cases of extreme debility where common sense might have been expected to prompt the conservancy of blood and strength as life-saving measures. Even the great Boerhaave prescribed copious and repeated bleedings in cases of advanced phthisis. Against this indiscriminate and excessive phlebotomy Wesley most sternly set his face.

Considering all these things we may perceive that Wesley, in his indictment of the medical profession on the score of 'theories

in a cure for the bite of a mad dog as saying he 'never knew this fail'. 'But it has sometimes failed', counters Wesley. He recognizes measles as one of the most lethal of children's diseases on account of chest complications, advises 'for some weeks take care of catching cold', and recommends, 'Immediately consult an honest physician'.

For the most part Wesley has avoided remedies prepared from unpleasant sources. Exceptions to this are found where goose dung is mixed with celandine to cleanse and heal an ulcerating breast, where dried human dung is finely powdered to blow into the eye for the cure of 'films', and where cow dung strewn with cummin seeds is applied as a hot, thick plaster spread on leather in cases of windy rupture. In contrast, a great many of the eighteenth-century cures were derived from most curious and unpleasant sources. The *New London Dispensatory* with unsavoury thoroughness searches every possible source for its medicaments—the juice of pounded lice, powders from human hair and nails, chameleon dung mixed with apes' urine.

Some affinities in treatment between those days and ours may be noted. For quinsey of the breast, 'A sudden unaccountable pain and difficulty of breathing seizing a person in the night or on any violent motion'—that is to say a coronary thrombosis—Wesley gave laudanum; today, opium's derivative morphine is prescribed. The value of a diet of turnips and nettle juice every morning, not to mention the juice of Seville oranges, would remain good specific treatment for scurvy today. With regard to St Anthony's Fire—erysipelas—we have to confess that until the advent of the sulphonamides our suggestions for cure were no better than those contained in *Primitive Physic*.

Some otherwise unknown names are here immortalized. Mr Masters of Evesham was a patient of Doctor Dover (of Dover's Powder fame) and was 'far gone in consumption'. Dr Dover advised him to lose six ounces of blood every day for a fortnight, if he lived so long, and then every other day: then every third day; then every fifth day. In three months he was well! Mrs Bates (No. 26) and Mrs Watts (No. 44) are two other such names. With their multiple ailments they belong to a type of patient that has not passed with the eighteenth century. Mrs

Bates was afflicted with cancer, consumption, sciatica and rheumatism for 'near twenty years'. Mrs Watts suffered from hysteric colic, fits, sweatings, vomitings, wandering pains, total loss of appetite. Today we should treat Mrs Bates and Mrs Watts from a wide range of tranquillizing tablets. Which of us would have the courage to order for them a cold bath every morning, and which of us could display such an authority as would ensure its punctual use until the ladies were driven from the thicket of their symptoms into an uncomplaining normality?

Wesley had much faith in cold bathing, partly, maybe, with an eye upon its subsidiary cleansing effect. His first cure for raging madness is to try the cooling effect of 'head cloths dipt in cold water'. His next-in-order cure is to place the patient 'with his head under a great water-fall as long as his strength will bear'. This moves towards a more drastic form of treatment. No mere cooling effect is now sought. The waterfall is a 'great' one, and the patient is held in position till breaking-point—'as long as his strength will bear'. This belongs to the category o shock treatment. Here is something in lineal descent from th old, cruel whippings at Bedlam, which were so often followed by behaviour improvement. It is humanized and controlled in modern shock therapy, whether by insulin or electric current, but the principle is the same. It is carried out just over the margin of endurance that it may be effective.

A large optimism pervades Wesley's presentation of these remedies. He has an ingenious cure for a cold in the head; he does not shrink from the problem of baldness or an old stubborn pain in the back; and he has encouraging words for old age. He ranges over a wide variety of illnesses, from abortion and ague to whitlows and worms. The sophisticated and well, those who are whole and need not a physician, may see in many of these remedies small ground for his optimism. But Wesley is no dilettante exhibiting his skill, or cheapjack parading his wares. He is the earnest healer entering the homes of thousands of ailing people; and what use if he does not enter with an infectious assurance that renews faith and hope, and rekindles natural healing processes? This optimism was justified by the popularity of his little book over so many years and through so many editions.   Doctor William Buchan, with some success, rode on the tide of this popularity in his book *Domestic Medicine*, which was largely an elaborated copy—though unacknowledged—of *Primitive Physic*.

Wesley's optimism reaches high-water-mark when he comes to espouse the curative value of electricity: 'Certainly it comes the nearest to a universal medicine of any yet known in the world', especially, he says elsewhere, in nervous cases.   Here we must remember that this is the enthusiasm natural and necessary to a pioneer battling against opposition and using his new friction machine in uncharted fields.   Wesley and Robert Lovett were the first two who made a serious attempt to use electricity in medicine and their names should not be forgotten.

We see Wesley as a pioneer in electric therapy and in hygiene and preventive medicine, but, even more important, we see him in these simple remedies setting an example and pointing the way out of obfuscating theories and pompous humbug to a rational approach to healing, to experiment and experience, to primitive physic.   We see him as a beneficent being, exercising a national influence and guiding medicine into ever-widening streams of usefulness to mankind.

A. WESLEY HILL

WREXHAM
August 1960

Additional notes and corrections are enclosed in square brackets.

A.W.H.

PRIMITIVE PHYSIC:

OR

An EASY and NATURAL METHOD

OF

C U R I N G

MOST

DISEASES

By JOHN WESLEY, M.A.

Homo sum: humani nihil a me alienum puto.

THE TWENTY-THIRD EDITION

L O N D O N:

Printed and sold at the New-Chapel, City-Road; and at
the Rev. Mr. WESLEY's Preaching Houses in Town
and Country. 1791.

THE

PREFACE

WHEN man came first out of the hands of the great Creator, clothed in body as well as in soul, with immortality and incorruption, there was no place for physic, or the art of healing. As he knew no sin, so he knew no pain, no sickness, weakness, or bodily disorder. The habitation wherein the angelic mind, the *Divinæ Particula Auræ*, abode, although originally formed out of the dust of the earth, was liable to no decay. It had no seeds of corruption or dissolution within itself. And there was nothing without to injure it: heaven and earth and all the hosts of them were mild, benign and friendly to human nature. The entire creation was at peace with man, so long as man was at peace with his Creator. So that well might *the morning-stars sing together, and all the sons of* God *shout for joy*.

2. But since man rebelled against the Sovereign of heaven and earth, how entirely is the scene changed! The incorruptible frame hath put on corruption, the immortal has put on mortality. The seeds of weakness and pain, of sickness and death, are now lodged in our inmost substance; whence a thousand disorders continually spring, even without the aid of external violence. And how is the number of these increased by every thing round about us? The heavens, the earth, and all things contained therein, conspire to punish the rebels against their Creator. The sun and moon shed unwholesome influences from above; the earth exhales poisonous damps from beneath: the beasts of the field, the birds of the air, the fishes of the sea, are in a state of hostility: the air itself that surrounds us

on every side, is replete with the shafts of death: yea, the food we eat, daily saps the foundation of that life which cannot be sustained without it. So has the Lord of all secured the execution of his decree,—"*Dust thou art, and unto dust thou shalt return.*"

3. But can nothing be found to lessen those inconveniences, which cannot be wholly removed? To soften the evils of life, and prevent in part the sickness and pain to which we are continually exposed? Without question there may. One grand preventative of pain and sickness of various kinds, seems intimated by the grand Author of Nature in the very sentence that intails death upon us: "In the sweat of thy face shalt thou eat bread, till thou return to the ground." The power of exercise, both to preserve and restore health, is greater than can well be conceived: especially in those who add temperance thereto; who, if they do not confine themselves altogether to eat either "Bread or the herb of the Field" (which God does not require them to do), yet steadily observe both that kind and measure of food, which experience shews to be most friendly to health and strength.

4. It is probable Physic, as well as Religion, was in the first ages chiefly traditional: every father delivering down to his sons, what he had himself in like manner received, concerning the manner of healing both outward hurts, and the diseases incident to each climate, and the medicines which were of the greatest efficacy for the cure of each disorder. It is certain this is the method wherein the art of healing is preserved among the *Americans* to this day. Their diseases indeed are exceeding few; nor do they often occur by reason of their continual exercise, and (till of late) universal temperance. But if any are sick, or bit by a serpent, or torn by a wild beast, the fathers immediately tell their children what remedy to apply. And it is rare that the patient suffers long; those medicines being quick, as well as generally infallible.

5. Hence it was, perhaps, that the Ancients, not only of *Greece* and *Rome*, but even of barbarous nations, usually assigned physic a divine original. And indeed it was a natural thought, that He who had taught it to the very beasts and birds, the

24

Cretan Stag, the *Egyptian* Ibis, could not be wanting to teach man,

Sanctius his Animal, mentisque capacius altæ:

Yea, sometimes even by those meaner creatures: for it was easy to infer, "If this will heal that creature, whose flesh is nearly of the same texture with mine, then in a parallel case it will heal me." The trial was made: the cure was wrought: and Experience and Physic grew up together.

6. And has not the Author of Nature taught us the use of many other medicines, by what is vulgarly termed Accident? Thus one walking some years since in a grove of pines, at a time when many in the neighbouring town were afflicted with a kind of new distemper, little sores in the inside of the mouth, a drop of the natural gum fell from one of the trees on the book which he was reading. This he took up, and thoughtlessly applied to one of those sore places. Finding the pain immediately cease he applied it to another, which was also presently healed. The same remedy he afterwards imparted to others, and it did not fail to heal any that applied it. And doubtless numberless remedies have been thus casually discovered in every age and nation.

7. Thus far physic was wholly founded on experiment. The *European*, as well as the *American*, said to his neighbour, Are you sick? Drink the juice of this herb, and your sickness will be at an end. Are you in a burning heat? Leap into that river, and then sweat till you are well. Has the snake bitten you? Chew and apply that root, and the poison will not hurt you. Thus ancient men, having a little experience joined with common sense and common humanity, cured both themselves and their neighbours of most of the distempers, to which every nation was subject.

8. But in process of time, men of a philosophical turn were not satisfied with this. They began to enquire how they might *account* for these things? How such Medicines wrought such effects? They examined the human body, and all its parts; the nature of the flesh, veins, arteries, nerves; the structure of the brain, heart, lungs, stomach, bowels; with the springs of the

several kinds of animal functions. They explored the several kinds of animal and mineral, as well as vegetable substances. And hence the whole order of physic, which had obtained to that time, came gradually to be inverted. Men of learning began to set aside experience; to build physic upon hypothesis; to form theories of diseases and their cure, and to substitute these in the place of experiments.

9. As theories increased, simple medicines were more and more disregarded and disused: till in a course of years the greater part of them were forgotten, at least in the politer nations. In the room of these, abundance of new ones were introduced by reasoning, speculative men: and those more and more difficult to be applied, as being more remote from common observation. Hence rules for the application of these, and medical books were immensely multiplied; till at length physic became an abstruse science, quite out of the reach of ordinary men.

10. Physicians now began to be had in admiration, as persons who were somethng more than human. And profit attended their employ as well as honour; so that they had now two weighty reasons for keeping the bulk of mankind at a distance, that they might not pry into the mysteries of the profession. To this end, they increased those difficulties by design, which began in a manner by accident. They filled their writings with abundance of technical terms, utterly unintelligible to plain men. They affected to deliver their rules, and to reason upon them, in an abstruse and philosophical manner. They represented the critical knowledge of Astronomy, Natural Philosophy (and what not? Some of them insisting on that of Astronomy, and Astrology too) as necessarily previous to the understanding the art of healing. Those who understood only how to restore the sick to health, they branded with the name of Empirics. They introduced into practice abundance of compound medicines, consisting of so many ingredients, that it was scarce possible for common people to know which it was that wrought the cure: abundance of exotics, neither the nature nor names of which their own countrymen understood: of chymicals, such as they neither had skill, nor fortune, nor time to prepare: yea, and of dangerous ones, such as they could not use, without hazarding

life, but by the advice of a physician. And thus both their honour and gain were secured, a vast majority of mankind being utterly cut off from helping either themselves or their neighbours, or once daring to attempt it.

11. Yet there have not been wanting, from time to time, some lovers of mankind, who have endeavoured (even contrary to their own interest) to reduce physic to its ancient standard: who have laboured to explode it out of all the hypotheses, and fine spun theories, and to make it a plain intelligible thing, as it was in the beginning: having no more mystery in it than this, "Such a medicine removes such a pain." These have demonstrably shewn, That neither the knowledge of Astrology, Astronomy, Natural Philosophy, nor even Anatomy itself, is absolutely necessary to the quick and effectual cure of most diseases incident to human bodies: nor yet any chimical, or exotic, or compound medicine, but a single plant or root duly applied. So that every man of common sense (unless in some rare cases) may prescribe either to himself or his neighbour; and may be very secure from doing harm, even where he can do no good.

12. Even in the last age there was something of this kind done, particularly by the great and good Dr. *Sydenham:* and in the present, by his pupil Dr. *Dover,* who has pointed out simple medicines for many diseases. And some such may be found in the writings of the learned and ingenious Dr. *Cheyne:* who doubtless would have communicated many more to the world, but for the melancholy reason he gave one of his friends, that prest him with some passages in his works, which too much countenanced the modern practice, "O Sir, we must do something *to oblige the Faculty,* or they will tear us in pieces."

13. Without any regard to this, without any concern about the obliging or disobliging any man living, a mean hand has made here some little attempt towards a plain and easy way of curing most diseases. I have only consulted herein, Experience, Common Sense, and the common Interest of mankind. And supposing they can be cured this easy way, who would desire to use any other? Who would not wish to have a Physician always in his house, and one that attends without fee or reward?

To be able (unless in some few complicated cases) to prescribe to his family, as well as himself?

14. If it be said, but what need is there of such attempt? I answer, the greatest that can possibly be conceived. Is it not needful in the highest degree, to rescue men from the jaws of destruction? From wasting their fortunes, as thousands have done, and continue to do daily? From pining away in sickness and pain, either through the ignorance or dishonesty of Physicians? Yea, and many times throwing away their lives, after their health, time and substance?

Is it enquired, but are there not books enough already, on every part of the art of medicine? Yes, too many ten times over, considering how little to the purpose the far greater part of them speak. But beside this, they are too dear for poor men to buy, and too hard for plain men to understand. Do you say, "But there are enough of these collections of Receipts." Where? I have not seen one yet, either in our own or any other tongue, which contains only safe, and cheap, and easy medicines. In all that have yet fallen into my hand, I find many dear and many far-fetched medicines: besides many of so dangerous a kind, as a prudent man would never meddle with. And against the greater part of those medicines there is a further objection: they consist of too many ingredients. The common method of compounding and de-compounding medicines, can never be reconciled to Common Sense. Experience shews, that one thing will cure most disorders, at least as well as twenty put together. Then why do you add the other nineteen? Only to swell the Apothecary's bill: nay, possibly, on purpose to prolong the distemper, that the Doctor and he may divide the spoil.

But admitting there is some quality in the medicine proposed which has need to be *corrected*; will not one thing correct it as well as twenty? It is probable, much better. And if not, there is a sufficiency of other medicines, which need no such correction.

How often, by thus compounding medicines of opposite qualities, is the virtue of both utterly destroyed? Nay, how often do those joined together destroy life, which single might have preserved it? This occasioned that caution of the great *Boerha[a]ve*, against mixing things without evident necessity, and without full proof of the effect they will produce when joined together, as well as of that they produce when asunder: seeing (as he observes) several things, which separately taken, are safe and powerful medicines, when compounded, not only lose their former powers, but commence a strong and deadly poison.

15. As to the manner of using the medicines here set down, I should advise, As soon as you know your distemper, (which is very easy, unless in a complication of disorders, and then you would do well to apply to a Physician that fears God:) *First*, use the first of the remedies for that disease which occurs in the ensuing collection; (unless some other of them be easier to be had, and then it may do just as well.) *Secondly*, After a competant time, if it takes no effect, use the second, the third, and so on. I have purposely set down (in most cases) several remedies for each disorder; not only because all are not equally easy to be procured at all times, and in all places: but likewise because the medicine which cures one man, will not always cure another of the same distemper. Nor will it cure the same man at all times. Therefore it was necessary to have a variety. However, I have subjoined the letter (*I*) to those medicines which some think to be *Infallible*.——*Thirdly*, Observe all the time the greatest exactness in your regimen or manner of living. Abstain from all mixed, all high-seasoned food. Use plain diet, easy of digestion; and this as sparingly as you can, consistent with ease and strength. Drink only water, if it agrees with your stomach; if not, good clear, small beer. Use as much exercise daily in the open air as you can without weariness. Sup at six or seven, on the lightest food: go to bed early, and rise betimes. To persevere with steadiness in this course, is often more than half the cure. Above all, add to the rest, (for it is not labour lost) that old unfashionable Medicine, Prayer. And have faith in God who "*killeth and maketh alive, who bringeth down to the grave, and bringeth up.*"

16. For the sake of those who desire, through the blessing of God, to retain the health which they have recovered, I have added a few plain, easy Rules, chiefly transcribed from Dr. *Cheyne*.

I. 1. *The air* we breathe is of great consequence to our health. Those who have been long abroad in Easterly or Northerly winds, should drink some thin and warm Liquor going to bed, or a draught of toast and water.

2. Tender people should have those who lie with them, or are much about them, sound, sweet, and healthy.

3. Every one that would preserve health, should be as clean and sweet as possible in their houses, clothes and furniture.

II. 1. The great rule of *eating and drinking* is, To suit the quality and quantity of the food to the strength of our digestion; to take always such a sort and such a measure of food as fits light and easy to the stomach.

2. All pickled, or smoaked, or salted food, and all high-seasoned is unwholesome.

3. Nothing conduces more to health, than abstinence and plain food, with due labour.

4. For studious persons, about eight ounces of animal food, and twelve of vegetable in twenty-four hours is sufficient.

5. Water is the wholesomest of all drinks; quickens the appetite, and strengthens the digestion most.

6. Strong, and more especially spirituous liquors, are a certain, though slow, poison.

7. Experience shews, there is very seldom any danger in leaving them off all at once.

8. Strong liquors do not prevent the mischiefs of a surfeit, nor carry it off so safely as water.

9. Malt liquors (except clear, small beer, or small ale, of due age) are exceeding hurtful to tender persons.

10. Coffee and tea are extremely hurtful to persons who have weak nerves.

III. 1. Tender persons should eat very light suppers; and that two or three hours before going to bed.

2. They ought constantly to go to bed about nine, and rise at four or five.

IV. 1. A due degree of *exercise* is indispensably necessary to health and long life.

2. Walking is the best exercise for those who are able to bear

it; riding for those who are not. The open air, when the weather is fair, contributes much to the benefit of exercise.

3. We may strengthen any weak part of the body by constant exercise. Thus the lungs may be strengthened by loud speaking, or walking up an easy ascent; the digestion and the nerves, by riding; the arms and hams, by strongly rubbing them daily.

4. The studious ought to have stated times for exercise, at least two or three hours a-day: the one half of this before dinner, the other before going to bed.

5. They should frequently shave, and frequently wash their feet.

6. Those who read or write much, should learn to do it standing; otherwise it will impair their health.

7. The fewer clothes any one uses, by day or night, the hardier he will be.

8. Exercise, first, should be always on an empty stomach; secondly, should never be continued to weariness; thirdly, after it, we should take care to cool by degrees; otherwise we shall catch cold.

9. The flesh brush is a most useful exercise, especially to strengthen any part that is weak.

10. Cold-bathing is of great advantage to health: it prevents abundance of diseases. It promotes perspiration, helps the circulation of the blood, and prevents the danger of catching cold. Tender people should pour water upon the head before they go in, and walk swiftly. To jump in with the head foremost, is too great a shock to nature.

V. 1. Costiveness cannot long conflict with health. Therefore care should be taken to remove it at the beginning: and, when it is removed, to prevent its return, by soft, cool, opening diet.

2. Obstructed perspiration (vulgarly called catching cold) is one great source of diseases. Whenever there appears the least sign of this, let it be removed by gentle sweats.

VI. 1. *The passions* have a greater influence on health, than most people are aware of.

2. All violent and sudden passions dispose to, or actually throw people into acute diseases.

3. The slow and lasting passions, such as grief and hopeless love, bring on chronical diseases.

4. Till the passion, which caused the disease, is calmed, medicine is applied in vain.

5. The love of God, as it is the sovereign remedy of all miseries, so in particular it effectually prevents all the bodily disorders the passions introduce, by keeping the passions themselves within due bounds. And by the unspeakable joy and perfect calm, serenity, and tranquility it gives the mind, it becomes the most powerful of all the means of health and long life.

LONDON, *June* 11, 1747.

POSTSCRIPT

1. IT was a great surprise to the Editor of the following Collection, that there was so swift and large a demand for it; that three impressions were called for in four or five years; and that it was not only re-published by the Booksellers of a neighbouring nation; but also inserted by parts in their public papers, and so propagated through the whole kingdom. This encouraged him carefully to revise the whole, and to publish it again, with several alterations, which it is hoped may make it of greater use to those who love common sense and common honesty.

2. Those alterations are still in pursuance of my first design, to set down cheap, safe, and easy medicines; easy to be known, easy to be procured, and easy to be applied by plain, unlettered men. Accordingly, I have omitted a considerable number, which though cheap and safe, were not so common or well known; and have added at least an equal number, to which that objection cannot be made: which are not only of small price, and extremely safe, but likewise easily to be found, if not in every house or yard, yet in every town, and almost every village throughout the kingdom.

3. It is because they are not safe, but extremely dangerous, that I have omitted (together with Antimony) the four *Herculean* medicines, Opium,* the Bark,* Steel,* and most of the preparations of Quicksilver. *Herculean* indeed! Far too strong for common men to grapple with. How many fatal effects have these produced even in the hands of no ordinary Physicians! With regard to four of these, the instances are glaring and undeniable. And whereas Quicksilver, the fifth, is in its native form as innocent as bread or water: has not the art been discovered, so to *prepare* it, as to make it the most deadly of all poisons? *These*, Physicians have justly termed edged Tools.

* Except in a very few Cases.

But they have not yet taught them to wound at a distance: and honest men are under no necessity of touching them, or coming within their reach.

4. Instead of these, I have once more ventured to recommend to men of plain, unbiassed reason, such remedies as air, water, milk, whey, honey, treacle, salt, vinegar, and common *English* herbs, with a few foreign medicines, almost equally cheap, safe and common. And this I have done on that principle, whereby I desire to be governed in all my actions, "*Whatsoever ye would that men should do unto you, the same do unto them.*"

5. At the request of many persons, I have likewise added plain definitions of most distempers; not indeed accurate or philosophical definitions, but such as are suited to men of ordinary capacities, and as may just enable them, in common simple cases, to distinguish one disease from another. In uncommon or complicated diseases, where life is more immediately in danger, I again advise every man without delay to apply to a Physician that fears God.

BRISTOL, *Oct.* 16, 1755.

London, Nov. 10, 1760.

DURING the observation and experience of more than five years, which have passed since the last impression of this Tract, I have had many opportunities of trying the virtues of the ensuing Remedies. And I have now added the word *Tried* to those which I have found to be of the greatest efficacy. I believe many others to be of equal virtue: but it has not lain in my way to make the trial.

In this course of time I have likewise had occasion to collect several other Remedies, tried either by myself or others, which are inserted under their proper heads. Some of these I have found to be of uncommon virtue, equal to any of those which were before published: and one, I must aver, from personal knowledge, grounded on a thousand experiments, to be far superior to all the other medicines I have known; I mean *Electricity*. I cannot but intreat all those who are well-wishers

34

to mankind, to make full proof of this. Certainly it comes the nearest an universal medicine, of any yet known in the world.

One grand advantage which most of these medicines have above those commonly used is this; you may be sure of having them good in their kind; pure, genuine, unsophisticate. But who can be sure of this, when the medicines he uses are compounded by an Apothecary? Perhaps he has not the drug prescribed by the Physician, and so puts in its place "what will do as well." Perhaps he has it; but it is stale and perished: yet "you would not have him throw it away. Indeed he cannot afford it." Perhaps he cannot afford to make up the medicine as the Dispensatory directs, and sell it at the common price. So he puts in cheaper ingredients: and you take neither you nor the Physician knows what! How many inconveniencies must this occasion! How many constitutions are ruined hereby! How many valuable lives are lost! Whereas all these inconveniencies may be prevented, by a little care and common sense, in the use of those plain, simple Remedies, which are here collected.

Otley, April 20, 1780.

SINCE the last Correction of this Tract, near twenty years ago, abundance of objections have been made to several parts of it. These I have considered with all the attention which I was master of: and in consequence hereof, have now omitted many Articles, and altered many others. I have likewise added a considerable number of Medicines, several of which have been but lately discovered: and several (although they had been long in use) I had never tried before. But I still advise, "in complicated cases, or where life is in immediate danger, let every one apply without delay, to a Physician that fears God." From one who does not, be his fame ever so great, I should expect a curse rather than a blessing.

⁎ Most of those Medicines which I prefer to the rest, are now marked with an Asterisk.

A COLLECTION OF
RECEIPTS

1. *Abortion, (to prevent.)*

1. WOMEN of a weak or relaxed habit should use solid food, avoiding great quantities of tea, and other weak, and watery liquors. They should go soon to bed, and rise early; and take frequent exercise, but avoid being over-fatigued.

2. If of a full habit, they ought to use a spare diet, and chiefly of the vegetable kind, avoiding strong liquors, and every thing that may tend to heat the body, or increase the quantity of blood.

In the first case, take daily half a pint of decoction of *Lignum Guaiacum;* boiling an ounce of it in a quart of water for five minutes.

In the latter case, give half a drachm of powdered *Nitre*, in a cup of water-gruel, every five or six hours: in both cases she should sleep on a hard mattress with her head low, and be kept cool and quiet.

2. *For an Ague.**

3. Go into the *Cold-Bath* just before the cold fit.

☞ *Nothing tends more to prolong an Ague, than indulging a lazy indolent disposition. The patient ought therefore between the fits to take as much exercise as he can bear; and to use a light diet, and for common drink,* Lemonade *is the most proper.*

---

* An *Ague* is, An Intermitting Fever, each fit of which is preceded by a cold shivering, and goes off in a sweat.

When all other means fail, give *blue Vitriol*, from one grain to two grains, in the absence of the fit; and repeat it three or four times in twenty-four hours:

4. Or, take a handful of *Groundsell*, shred it small, put it into a paper-bag, four Inches square, pricking that side which is to be next the skin full of holes. Cover this with a thin linen, and wear it on the pit of the stomach, renewing it two hours before the fit: Tried.

5. Or, apply to the stomach, a large *Onion* slit:

☞ 6. Or, melt two-penny worth of *Frankincense*, spread it on linen, grate a *Nutmeg* upon it, cover it with linen, and hang this bag on the pit of the stomach.—I have never yet known it fail:

7. Or, boil *Yarrow* in new milk, till it is tender enough to spread as a plaister. An hour before the cold fit, apply this to the wrists, and let it be on till the hot fit is over. If another fit comes, use a fresh plaister.—This often cures a *Quartan*.

8. Or, drink a quart of *cold water*, just before the cold fit. Then go to bed and sweat:

9. Or, make six middling pills of *Cobwebs*. Take one a little before the cold fit: two a little before the next fit: (suppose the next day:) the other three, if needs be, a little before the third fit. This seldom fails:—Or, put a tea-spoonful of *Salt of Tartar* into a large glass of spring water, and drink it by little and little. Repeat the same dose the next two days, before the time of the fit:

10. Or, two small tea-spoonfuls of *Sal Prunellæ*, an hour before the fit.—It commonly cures in thrice taking:

11. Or, a large spoonful of powdered *Camomile Flowers:*

*12. Or, a tea-spoonful of *Spirits of Hartshorn*, in a glass of water.

13. Or, eat a small *Lemon*, rind and all:

14. In the hot fit, if violent, take eight or ten drops of *Laudanum:* if costive, in *Hierapicra* ['Holy Bitters', a powder of Aloes and Canella].

37

15. Dr. *Lind* says, an *Ague* is certainly cured, by taking from ten to twenty drops of *Laudanum*, with two drachms of *Syrrup of Poppies* in any warm liquid, half an hour after the heat begins.

☞ *It is proper to take a gentle vomit, and sometimes a purge, before you use any of these medicines. If a vomit is taken two hours before the Fit is expected, it generally prevents that Fit, and sometimes cures an Ague: especially in children. —It is also proper to repeat the medicine (whatever it be) about a week after, in order to prevent a relapse. Do not take any purge soon after.——The daily use of the Flesh Brush,[1] and frequent cold bathing are of great use to prevent relapses.*

16. Children have been cured by wearing a waistcoat, in which *Bark*[2] was quilted.

3. *A Tertian Ague.**

17. Is often cured by taking a *purge* one day; and the next, *bleeding* in the beginning of the Fit:

18. Or, take a tea-spoonful of *Salt of Tartar* in spring-water. This often cures double Tertians, triple Quartans, and long lasting Fevers: especially if *Sena* be premised twice or thrice:

*19. Or apply to each wrist a plaister of *treacle* and *soot*.— Tried.

20. Or, use the *cold-bath*. (Unless you are of an advanced age, or extremely weak.) But when you use this, on any account whatever, it is proper,

1. To bleed or purge, before you begin:

2. To go in cool; to immerge at once, but not head-fore-most; to stay in only two or three minutes, or less, at first:

3. Never to bathe on a full stomach:

4. To bathe twice or thrice a week at least, till you have bathed nine or ten times:

* That is, An *Ague* which returns every other day.

[1 A soft brush to be used on the skin to promote circulation and excite the surface secretions. (*Lloyd's Encyclopaedic Dictionary*.)]

[2 He refers to Peruvian bark. Wesley was prejudiced against the Bark taken internally. See *Journal of John Wesley* (Standard Edition), IV. 91.]

5. To sweat immediately after it (going to bed) in palsies, rickets, and all diseases wherein the nerves are obstructed:

6. You may use yourself to it, without any danger, by beginning in *May*, and at first just plunging in, and coming out immediately. But many have begun in winter without any inconvenience.

4. *A Double Tertian.*

21. Take before the fit, (after a purge or two) three ounces of *Cichory-Water*, half a drachm of *Salt of Tartar*, and fifteen drops of *Spirit of Sulphur:*

22. To perfect the cure, on the fourth day after you miss the Fit, take two drachms of *Sena*, half a drachm of *Salt of Tartar*, infused all night in four ounces of *Cichory-Water*. Strain it and drink it.

5. *A Quartan Ague.**

23. Apply to the suture of the head, when the fit is coming, *Wall July Flowers*, beating together leaves and flowers with a little salt. Keep it on till the hot fit is over. Repeat this, if need be.

24. Use *strong exercise*, (as riding or walking, as far as you can bear it) an hour or two before the fit. If possible, continue it till the fit begins. This alone will frequently cure:—Tried.

25. Or, apply to the wrists a plaister of *Turpentine:* or, of bruised *Pepper*, mixt with *Treacle*.

26. Or, apply *oil of turpentine* to the small of the back, before the fit.

27. For a *Tertian* or *Quartan*, vomit with ten grains of Ipecacuanha an hour before the cold fit begins. Then go to bed, and continue a large sweat by *lemonade*, (that is, lemon, sugar, and water) for six or eight hours. This usually cures in three or four times. If it does not, use the *cold-bath* between the fits.

* That is, An *Ague* which misses two days; coming on *Monday* (suppose) and again on *Thursday*.

28. Or, take twenty grains of powdered *Saffron* before the fit, in a glass of white wine.

6. *St. Anthony's Fire** [*Erysipelas*].

*29. Take a glass of *tar-water* warm in bed, every hour, washing the part with the same.

☞ Tar-water *is made thus.—Put a gallon of cold water to a quart of Norway tar. Stir them together with a flat stick for five or six minutes. After it has stood covered for three days, pour off the water clear, bottle and cork it.*

*30. Or, take a decoction of *elder leaves*, as a sweat; applying to the part a cloth dipt in *lime-water*, mixed with a little *camphorated spirit of wine*.

☞ Lime-water *is made thus.——Infuse a pound of good quick lime in six quarts of spring-water for twenty-four hours. Decant and keep it for use.*

31. Or, take two or three gentle purges.—No acute Fever bears repeated purges better than this, especially when it affects the head: mean time boil a handful of *Sago*, two handfuls of *elder leaves* (or *bark*) and an ounce of *Alum* in two quarts of forge water, to a pint. Wash with this every night.—See Extract from Dr. *Tissot*, page 104.

32. If the pulse be low, and the spirits sunk, nourishing broths and a little negus may be given *to advantage*.

33. Or, let three drachms of *nitre* be dissolved in as much *elder-flower tea*, as the patient can drink in twenty-four hours. If the disease attacks the head, bleeding is necessary.

Dressing the inflammation with greasy ointments, salves, &c. is very improper.

34. Bathing the feet and legs in *warm water* is serviceable, and often relieves the patient much.—In Scotland the

---

* St. *Anthony's Fire* is a Fever attended with a red and painful swelling, full of *pimples*, which afterwards turn into *small blisters*, on the face or some other part of the body. The sooner the eruption is, the less danger. Let your diet be only *Water-Gruel*, or *Barley-Broth*, with roasted Apples.

common people cover the part with a linen cloth covered
with meal.

7. *The Apoplexy.*†

35. To prevent, use the *cold-bath*, and drink only water.

*36. In the fit, put a handful of *salt* into a pint of cold water,
and if possible, pour it down the throat of the patient.
He will quickly come to himself.   So will one who seems
dead by a fall.   But send for a good Physician immediately.

*37. If the fit be soon after a meal, do not bleed, but vomit.

*38. Rub the head, feet, and hands strongly, and let two
strong men carry the patient upright, backward and for-
ward about the room.

39. A *Seton* in the neck, with low diet, has often prevented
a relapse.——See Extract from Dr. *Tissot*, page 53.

There is a wide difference between the *Sanguineous*, and
Serous Apoplexy; the latter is often followed by a palsy.——
The former is distinguished by the countenance appear-
ing florid; the face swelled or puffed up; and the blood-
vessels, especially about the neck and temples, are turgid;
the pulse beats strong; the eyes are prominent and fixed;
and the breathing is difficult, and performed with a snorting.   This invades more suddenly than the Serous
Apoplexy.   Use large bleedings, from the arm, or neck;
bathe the feet in warm water; cupping on the back of the
head, with deep scarification.   The garters should be
tied very tight to lesson the motion of the blood from the
lower extremities.

A scruple of *Nitre* may be given in water, every three or
four hours.

When the patient is so far recovered as to be able to swallow,
let him take a strong purge; but if this cannot be effected,
a glyster[1] should be thrown up with plenty of fresh butter,
and a large spoonful of common salt in it.

† An *Apoplexy* is, a total loss of all sense, and voluntary motion, commonly attended with a strong pulse, hard breathing and snorting.

[[1] Glyster or clyster is an enema.]

In the *Serous Apoplexy*, the pulse is not so strong, the countenance is less florid, and not attended with so great a difficulty of breathing. Here bleeding is not so necessary, but a vomit of three grains of *Emetic Tartar* may be given, and afterwards a purge as before, and the powder of *white Hellebore* blown up the nose, &c.

☞ *This Apoplexy is generally preceded by an unusual heaviness, giddiness, and drowsiness.*

8. *Canine Appetite.*†

40. "If it be without vomiting, is often cured by a small bit of bread dipt in wine, and applied to the nostrils." *Dr. Schomberg.*

9. *The Asthma.*‡

41. Take a pint of *cold water* every morning washing the head therein immediately after, and using the *cold bath* once a fortnight.

*42. Or, cut an ounce of stick *Liquorice* into slices. Steep this in a quart of water, four and twenty hours, and use it, when you are worse than usual, as common drink. I have known this give much ease.

43. Or, half a pint of *Tar-Water*, twice a day.

44. Or, live a fortnight on boiled *Carrots* only. It seldom fails:

*45. Or, take an ounce of *Quicksilver* every morning, and a spoonful of *Aqua Sulphurata*, or fifteen drops of *Elixir of Vitriol*, in a large glass of spring-water at five in the evening.——This has cured an inveterate *Asthma*.

46. Or, take from ten to sixty drops of *Elixir of Vitriol*, in a glass of water, three or four times a day.

☞ Elixir of Vitriol *is made thus—Drop gradually four ounces of strong oil of vitriol into a pint of spirits of wine, or brandy:*

† An insatiable desire of eating.
‡ An *Asthma* is a difficulty of breathing from a disorder in the lungs. In the common (or moist) *Asthma*, the patient spits much.

let it stand three days, and add to it Ginger sliced, half an ounce, and Jamaica pepper, whole, one ounce. In three days more it is fit for use. But if the patient be subject to sour belchings, take the mixture for the Asthmatic cough, (as Art. 56 [57],*) after the Elixir of Vitriol.*

47. Or, into a quart of *boiling water,* put a teaspoonful of *Balsamic Æther,* receive the steam into the lungs, through a fumigater, twice a day.

☞ Balsamic Æther *is made thus.—Put four ounces of spirits of wine, and one ounce of Balsam of Tolu, into a vial, with one ounce of Æther. Keep it well corked. But it will not keep above a week.*

48. For present relief, vomit with a quart or more of *warm water.* The more you drink of it the better.

☞ *Do this whenever you find any motion to vomit; and take care always to keep your body open.*

10. *A Dry or Conclusive Asthma.*

49. Juice of *Radishes* relieve much: so does a cup of strong coffee: or, *Garlick,* either raw, or preserved, or in syrup:

50. Or, drink a pint of *New Milk* morning and evening.— This has cured an inveterate *Asthma.*

*51. Or, beat fine *Saffron* small, and take eight or ten grains every night.—Tried.

*52. Take from three to five grains of *Ipecacuanha* every morning; or from five to ten grains every other evening. Do this, if need be, for a month or six weeks. Five grains usually vomit. In a violent fit, take a scruple instantly.

53. In any *Asthma,* the best drink is *Apple Water:* that is, boiling water poured on sliced apples.

54. The food should be light and easy of digestion. *Ripe Fruits* baked, boiled, or roasted, are very proper; but strong liquors of all kinds, especially beer or ale are hurtful. If any supper is taken, it should be very light.

55. All disorders of the breast are much relieved by keeping the *feet warm*, and promoting perspiration. *Exercise* is also of very great importance; so that the patient should take as much every day, as his strength will bear. *Issues*[1] are found, in general, to be of great service.

56. Dr. *Smyth*, in his FORMULÆ, recommends *Mustard-Whey* as common drink, in the moist Asthma: and a decoction of the *Madder Root*, to promote spitting.

☞ The decoction is made thus.—*Boil an ounce of Madder, and two drachms of Mace, in three pints of water, to two pints, then strain it, and take a tea-cupful three or four times a day. But the most efficacious medicine is the* Quick-silver *and* Aqua Sulphurata. (as ART. [No.] 45.)—N.B. *Where the latter cannot be got, ten drops of* Oil of Vitriol, *in a large glass of spring water, will answer the same end.*—I have known many persons greatly relieved, and some cured, by taking as much *Jallop* [Jalap] every morning as would lie on a sixpence.

11. *To cure Baldness.*

57. Rub the part morning and evening, with *onions*, till it is red; and rub it afterwards with *honey*. Or, wash it with a decoction of *Boxwood:* Tried. Or, electrify it daily.

12. *Bleeding at the Nose, (to prevent.)*

*58. Drink *Whey* largely, every morning, and eat much *Raisins:*

59. Or, dissolve two scruples of *Nitre* in half a pint of water, and take a tea-cupful every hour.

60. To cure it, apply to the neck behind, and on each side, a cloth dipt in *cold water*.

61. Or, put the legs and arms in *cold water:*

*62. Or, wash the temples, nose, and neck with *vinegar:*

63. Or, keep a little roll of *white paper* under the tongue:

64. Or snuff up *vinegar* and *water:*[2]

[1 Issue—A suppurating sore made and kept open by inserting an irritant substance, say a pellet of orris root.]

[2 See *Journal of John Wesley* (Standard Edn), IV.113–14.]

65. Or, foment the legs and arms with it:

66. Or, steep a *linen rag* in *sharp vinegar*, burn it, and blow it up the nose with a quill:

67. Or, apply *Tents* made of soft lint, dipped in *cold water*, strongly impregnated with *Tincture of Iron*, and introduced within the nostrils quite through to their posterior apertures. This method, Mr. *Hey* says, never failed him:

68. Or, dissolve an ounce of *Alum* powdered, in a pint of *vinegar:* apply a cloth, dipt in this, to the temples, steeping the feet in *warm water*.

69. In a violent case, go into a pond or river. Tried.—See Extract from Dr. *Tissot*.

13. *Bleeding of a Wound.*

70. Make two or three tight *Ligatures* toward the lower part of each joint; slacken them gradually:

71. Or, apply tops of *Nettles* bruised:

72. Or, strew on it the *ashes* of a linen rag, dipt in sharp *vinegar* and burnt:

*73. Or take ripe *puff-balls*. Break them warily, and save the powder. Strew this on the wound and bind it on. *I*—This will stop the bleeding of an imputed [amputated] limb without any cautery.

74. Or take of *brandy*, two ounces, *Castile-soap*, two drachms, *Pot-ash*, one drachm. Scrape the soap fine and dissolve it in the brandy; then add the Pot-ash. Mix them well together, and keep them close stopt in a phial. Apply a little of this warmed to a bleeding vessel, and the blood immediately congeals.

14. *Spitting Blood.*

*75. Take a tea-cupful of stewed *prunes*, at lying down, for two or three nights: Tried.

45

*76. Or, two spoonfuls of juice of *nettles*, every morning, and a large cup of decoction of *nettles* at night, for a week: Tried.

77. Or, three spoonfuls of *sage-juice* in a little *honey*. This presently stops either spitting or vomiting blood: Tried.

78. Or, half a tea-spoonful of *Barbadoes tar*, on a lump of loaf sugar at night. It commonly cures at once.

15. *Vomiting Blood.*

*79. Take two spoonfuls of *nettle juice.*—

☞ (This also dissolves blood coagulated in the stomach.)— Tried.

80. Or, take as much *salt petre*, as will lie upon half a crown, dissolved in a glass of cold water, two or three times a day.

16. *To dissolve coagulated Blood.*

81. Bind on the part for some hours, a paste made of *black soap* and *crumbs of white bread:*

82. Or, grated root of *burdock* spread on a rag: renew this twice a day.

17. *Blisters.*

83. On the feet, occasioned by walking, are cured by drawing a needle full of *worsted* through them. Clip it off at both ends, and leave it till the skin peels off.

18. *Boils.*

84. Apply a little *Venice turpentine:*

85. Or, an equal quantity of *soap* and *brown sugar* well mixt:

86. Or, a plaister of *honey* and *wheat flower:*

87. Or, of *figs:*

88. Or, a little *saffron* in a white bread poultice.—'Tis proper to purge also.

19. *Hard Breasts.*

89. Apply *turnips roasted* till soft, then mashed and mixed with a little *oil of roses.* Change this twice a day, keeping the breast very warm with flannel.

20. *Sore Breasts and Swelled.*

*90. Boil a handful of *camomile* and as much *mallows* in milk and water. Foment with it between two flannels as hot as can be borne every twelve hours. It also dissolves any knot or swelling in any part.

21. *A Bruise.*

*91. Immediately apply *treacle* spread on brown paper: Tried.

92. Or, apply a plaister of chopt *parsley* mixt with butter:

*93. Or, *electrify* the part. This is the quickest cure of all.

22. *To prevent Swelling from a Bruise.*

94. Immediately apply a cloth, five or six times doubled, dipt in *cold water*, and new dipt when it grows warm: Tried.

23. *To cure a Swelling from a Bruise.*

95. Foment it half an hour, morning and evening with cloths dipped in *water* as hot as you can bear.

23. *A Burn or Scald.*

96. Immediately plunge the part into *cold water*. Keep it in an hour, if not well before. Perhaps four or five hours: Tried.

*97. Or, *electrify* it. If this can be done presently, it totally cures the most desperate burn.

98. Or, if the part cannot be dipt, apply a cloth four times doubled, dipt in *cold water*, changing it when it grows warm:

*99. Or, a bruised *onion:*

100. Or, apply *oil;* and strew on it powdered *ginger.*

47

25. *A deep Burn or Scald.*

101. Apply black *varnish* with a feather, till it is well:

102. Or, inner rind of *elder* well mixt with fresh butter. When this is bound on with a rag, plunge the part into cold water. This will suspend the pain, till the medicine heals.

103. Or, mix *lime-water* and *sweet oil*, to the thickness of cream, apply it with a feather, several times a day.—This is the most effectual application I ever met with:

104. Or put twenty-five drops of *Goullard's Extract of Lead*,[1] to half a pint of *rain water;* dip linen rags in it, and apply them to the part affected. This is particularly serviceable if the burn is near the eyes.

26. *A Cancer in the Breast.*†

*105. Of thirteen years standing, was cured by frequently applying *red poppy water, plantane,* and *rose water,* mixt with *honey of roses.* Afterwards, the waters used alone perfected the cure.

106. Use the *cold bath.* (This has cured many.) This cured Mrs. *Bates, of Leicestershire,* of a cancer in her breast, a consumption, a sciatica, and rheumatism, which she had had near twenty years. She bathed daily for a month, and drank only water.

A bleeding cancer was cured by drinking twice a day, a quarter of a pint of the juice of *clivers* or *goose-grass,* and covering the wounds with the bruised leaves.

[1 Extract of Saturn. Take 1 lb Letharge, 2 pints of Vinegar made of French wine. Put them together in a glazed earthen pipkin and let them simmer for an hour and a quarter, stirring them the while with a wooden spatula. After the whole has stood to settle, pour off the liquor which is upon the top into bottles for use.—Buchan's *Domestic Medicine*.]

† A *Cancer* is a hard, round, uneven, painful swelling, of a blackish or leaden colour, the veins round which seem ready to burst. It comes commonly with a swelling about as big as a pea, which does not at first give much pain, nor change the colour of the skin.

Another bleeding cancer was cured by the following receipt:

Take half a pint of *small beer*. When it boils, dissolve in it an ounce and a half of *bees-wax*. Then put in an ounce of *hogs-lard*, and boil them together. When it is cold, pour the *beer* from it, and apply it, spread upon white leather. Renew it every other day. It brings out great blotches, which are to be washed with *sal prunellæ* dissolved in warm water.

Monsieur *Le Febun* advises, "Dissolve four grains of *arsenic* in a pint of water. Take a spoonful of this, with a spoonful of *milk*, and half an ounce of *syrup of poppies*, every morning."

☞ *Generally where cold bathing is necessary to cure any disease, water-drinking is so, to prevent a relapse.*

107. If it be not broke, apply a piece of *sheet-lead*, beat very thin, and pricked full of pin-holes, for days or weeks, to the whole breast.——Purges should be added every third or fourth day.

108. Or, rub the whole breast morning and evening, with *spirits of hartshorn*, mixt with *oil*.

109. Or, keep it continually moist with honey.

*110. Or, take *horse spurs*† and dry them by the fire, till they will beat to powder. Sift and infuse two drachms in two quarts of ale: drink half a pint every six hours, new milk warm.——It has cured many: Tried.

111. Or, apply *goose dung* and *celandine*, beat well together and spread on a fine rag. It will both cleanse and heal the sore.

112. Or, a poultice of *wild parsnips*, flowers, leaves and stalks, changing it morning and evening: Or, scraped *carrots*:

113. Or, take *brimstone* [*quicksilver*] and *aqua sulphurata*. (See No. 45.)——This has cured one far advanced in years.——Dr. *Cheyne* says, a total Ass milk diet, about

† These are a kind of warts, that grow on the inside of the horse's fore-legs.

two quarts a day, without any other food or drink, will cure a confirmed cancer.

27. *A Cancer in any other Part.*

114. Apply red *onions* bruised:

115. Or, make a plaister of *roach-alum, vinegar,* and *honey,* equal quantities, with *wheat-flour.* Change it every twelve hours.—It often cures in three or four days:

116. Or stamp the flowers, leaves and stalks of wild *parsnips,* and apply them as a plaister, changing it every twelve hours.——It usually cures in a few days.

A Cancer under the eye was cured, by drinking a quart of *tar-water* daily, washing the same with it, and then applying a plaister of tar and mutton-suet melted together. It was well in two months, though of twenty years standing.

28. *A Cancer in the Mouth.*

117. Boil a few leaves of *succory, plantane,* and *rue,* with a spoonful of *honey,* for a quarter of an hour. Gargle with this often in an hour: *I.*

118. Or, with *vinegar* and *honey,* wherein half an ounce of *roche-alum* is boiled:

119. Or, mix as much burnt *alum* and as much black *pepper* as lies on a sixpence, with an ounce of *honey,* and frequently touch the part.

120. Or, blow the *ashes* of *scarlet* cloth into the mouth or throat. It seldom fails.

29. *Chilblains, (to prevent.)*

*121. Wear *flannel socks:* or, *socks* of *chamois leather.*

30. *Chilblains, (to cure.)*

122. Apply *salt* and *onions* pounded together:

*123. Or, a poultice of roasted *onions* hot. Keep it on two or three days, if not cured sooner.

50

124. Wash them (if broke) with tincture of *Myrrh* in a little water.—See Extract from Dr. *Tissot*.

31. *Children*.

125. To prevent the rickets, tenderness, and weakness, dip them in cold water every morning, at least till they are eight or nine months old.

No roller should ever be put round their bodies, nor any stays used. Instead of them, when they are put into short petticoats, put a waistcoat under their frocks.

Let them go bare-footed and bare-headed, till they are three or four years old at least.

'Tis best to wean a child when seven months old. It should lie in the cradle at least a year.

No child should touch any spirituous or fermented liquor, nor animal food, before two years old.

Their drink should be water. Tea they should never taste, till ten or twelve years old. Milk, milk porridge, and water-gruel, are the proper breakfasts for children.

32. *Chin-Cough, or Hooping-Cough*.

126. Use the *cold bath* daily.

127. Or, rub the feet thoroughly with *hogs-lard*, before the fire at going to bed, and keep the child warm therein: Tried.

128. Or, rub the back at lying down with *old rum*, It seldom fails.

129. Or, give a spoonful of juice of *penny-royal*, mixt with brown *sugar-candy*, twice a day:

130. Or, half a pint of *milk*, warm from the cow, with the quantity of a nutmeg of *conserve of roses* dissolved in it every morning.

*131. Or, dissolve a scruple of *salt of tartar* in a quarter of a pint of clear water: add to it ten grains of finely powdered *cochineal*, and sweeten it with loaf-sugar.

Give a child within the year, the fourth of a spoonful of this, four times a day, with a spoonful of barley-water after it. Give a child two years old, half a spoonful: a child above four years old a spoonful. Boiled apples put into warm milk may be his chief food. This relieves in twenty-four hours, and cures in five or six days.

132. Or, from three to five grains of *Gum Gamboge*.—It vomits and purges: and Dr. *Cook* says, always cures.

133. Or, take two grains of *tartar emetic*, and half a drachm of prepared *crabs claws*, powdered: let them be mixed very well together.

One grain, one grain and a half, or two grains of this composition, may be added to five or six grains of magnesia, and given in a small spoonful of milk and water in the forenoon between breakfast and dinner, to a child a year old.

At night, if the fever is very high, half the former dose of this powder may be given, with from five to ten grains of *nitre*.

134. In desperate cases, change of air alone has cured.

33. *Cholera Morbus: i.e. Flux and Vomiting.*

135. Drink two or three quarts of *cold water*, if strong; of *warm water*, if weak.

136. Or, boil a chicken an hour in two gallons of water, and drink of this till the vomiting ceases:

137. Or, decoction of *rice*, or *barley*, or toasted *oaten bread*.

If the pain is very severe, stupe the belly with flannels dipt in *spirits* and water.

The third day after the cure, take ten or fifteen grains of *rhubarb*.

34. *Chops in Women's Nipples.*

138. Apply *balsam of sugar*:

139. Or, apply *butter of wax*, which speedily heals them.

35. *Chopt Hands, (to prevent.)*

140. Wash them with *flour of mustard:*

141. Or, in *bran* and *water* boiled together.

(To Cure.)

*142. Wash with *soft soap*, mixed with *red sand:* tried.

143. Or, wash them in *sugar* and water: tried.

36. *Chopt Lips.*

144. Apply a little *sal prunella.*

37. *A Cold.*

*145. Drink a pint of *cold water* lying down in bed: tried.

146. Or, a spoonful of *treacle* in half a pint of water: tried.

147. Or, to one spoonful of *oatmeal*, and one spoonful of *honey*, add a piece of *butter*, the bigness of a nutmeg: pour on gradually near a pint of boiling water: drink this lying down in bed.

38. *A Cold in the Head.*

148. Pare very thin the *yellow rind* of an *orange*, roll it up inside out, and thrust a roll into each nostril.

39. *The Cholic (in the Fit.)*

*149. Drink a pint of *cold water:* tried.

150. Or, a quart of *warm water:* tried.

151. Or, of *camomile-tea;*

152. Or, take from thirty to forty grains of *yellow peel* of *oranges*, dried and powdered, in a glass of water:

153. Or, take from thirty to forty drops of *oil* of *aniseed* on a lump of sugar:

154. Or, apply outwardly a bag of *hot oats;*

155. Or, steep the legs in *hot water* a quarter of an hour:

156. Or, take as much *Daffy's Elixir* [see p. 121] as will presently purge. This relieves the most violent cholic in an hour or two.

40. *The Dry Cholic, (to prevent.)*

157. Drink *ginger tea.*

41. *Cholic in Children.*

158. Give a scruple of powdered *aniseed* in their meat: tried.

159. Or, small doses of *magnesia.*

160. Or put one grain of *emetic tartar* into six table-spoonfuls of *water;* a small tea-spoonful will puke a child of a week old; a large tea-spoonful is sufficient for one a month old; and so in proportion.—Repeat the puke every day, or every other day, as the case requires.

This is, perhaps, the best medicine yet discovered for infants. It speedily cures inward fits, gripes, looseness, thrush, and convulsions in children. But if the child is costive, his bowels must be opened first with a little magnesia, or manna, before you give a puke.

42. *Bilious Cholic.†*

161. Drink warm *lemonade:* I know nothing like it.

162. Or, give a spoonful of *sweet oil* every hour—This has cured one judged to be at the point of death.

43. *An Habitual Cholic.*

163. Wear a thin, soft flannel on the part.

44. *An Hysteric Cholic.‡*

164. Mrs. *Watts*, by using the *cold bath* two and twenty times in a month, was entirely cured of an hysteric cholic, fits,

† This is generally attended with vomiting a greenish or frothy matter, with feverish heat, violent thirst, a bitter taste in the mouth, and little and high-coloured urine.

‡ Is attended with a violent pain about the pit of the stomach, with great sinking of the spirits, and often with greenish vomitings.

and convulsive motions, continual sweatings and vomiting, wandering pains in her limbs and head, with total loss of appetite.

165. In the fit, drink half a pint of *water* with a little *wheat-flour* in it, and a spoonful of *vinegar*.

166. Or of warm *lemonade:* tried.

167. Or, take 20, 30, or 40 drops of *balsam* of *peru* on fine *sugar:* if need be, take this twice or thrice a day:

168. Or, in extremity, boil three ounces of *Burdock-seed* in water, which give as a clyster [enema]:

169. Or, twenty drops of *laudanum*, in any proper clyster, which gives instant ease.

45. *A Nervous Cholic.*†

170. Use the *cold-bath* daily for three or four weeks.

171. Or, take *quicksilver* and *aqua sulphurata* daily for a month: (as ART [No.] 45.)

46. *Cholic from the Fumes of Lead, or White Lead, Verdigrease, &c.*

172. In the fit, drink fresh *melted butter*, and then vomit with *warm water:*

173. To prevent or cure. Breakfast daily on *fat broth*, and use *oil of sweet almonds* frequently and largely.

174. Smelters of metals, plumbers, &c. may be in a good measure preserved from the poisonous fumes that surround them, by breathing through cloth or flannel mufflers twice or thrice doubled, dipt in a solution of *sea salt*, or *salt of tartar*, and then dried. These mufflers might also be of great use in similar cases.

† This some term the *dry belly-ach*. It often continues several days, with little urine, and obstinate costiveness.

A *cholic* with purging, some term the *watery gripes*.

175. *Parched peas* eaten freely, have had the most happy effect, when all other means have failed.

48. *To prevent the ill Effects of Cold.*

176. The moment a person gets into a house, with his hands or feet quite chilled, let him put them into a vessel of water, as cold as can be got, and hold them there till they begin to glow. This they will do in a minute or two. This method likewise effectually prevents chilblains.

49. *A Consumption.*

177. *Cold bathing* has cured many deep consumptions: tried.

178. One in a deep consumption was advised to drink nothing but *water*, and eat nothing but *water-gruel*, without salt or sugar. In three months time he was perfectly well.

179. Take no food but new *butter-milk*, churned in a bottle, and *white bread*.—I have known this successful.

180. Or, use as common drink, *spring-water*, and *new milk*, each a quart; and *sugar-candy* two ounces.

181. Or, boil two handfuls of *sorrel* in a pint of whey. Strain it, and drink a glass thrice a day: tried.

182. Or, turn a pint of skimmed milk with half a pint of small beer. Boil in this whey about twenty *ivy-leaves*, and two or three sprigs of *hyssop*. Drink half over night, the rest in the morning. Do this, if needful, for two months daily.——This has cured in a desperate case: tried.

183. Or, take a *cow-heel* from the tripe-house ready drest, two quarts of *new milk*, two ounces of *hartshorn shavings*, two ounces of *isinglass*, a quarter of a pound of *sugar-candy*, and a race of *ginger*. Put all these in a pot: and set them in an oven after the bread is drawn. Let it continue there till the oven is near cold; and let the patient live on

this.——I have known this cure a deep consumption more than once.

184. Or, every morning cut up a little turf of fresh earth, and lying down, breathe into the hole for a quarter of an hour.—I have known a deep consumption cured thus:

185. "Mr. *Masters*, of *Evesham*, was so far gone in a consumption, that he could not stand alone. I advised him to lose six ounces of blood every day for a fortnight, if he lived so long; and then every other day; then every third day; then every fifth day, for the same time. In three months he was well."——(Dr. *Dover*.) Tried.

186. Or, throw *frankincense* on burning coals, and receive the smoke daily through a proper tube into the lungs: tried.

187. Or, take in for a quarter of an hour, morning and evening, the steam of *white rosin* and *bees-wax*, boiling on a hot fire-shovel. This has cured one who was in the third stage of a consumption.

188. Or, the steam of sweet *spirit of vitriol* dropt into warm water:

189. Or, take morning and evening, a tea-spoonful of *white rosin* powdered and mixt with *honey*.—This cured one in less than a month, who was very near death.

190. Or, drink thrice a day two spoonfuls of juice of *water-cresses*.——This has cured a deep consumption.

191. In the last stage, *suck a healthy woman* daily. This cured my Father.

For diet, use *milk* and *apples*, or *water-gruel* made with fine flour. Drink *cyder-whey*, *barley-water*, sharpened with *lemon-juice*, or *apple-water*.

So long as the tickling cough continues, chew well and swallow a mouthful or two, of a biscuit or crust of bread, twice a day. If you cannot swallow it, spit it out. This will always shorten the fit, and would often prevent a consumption.—See Extract from Dr. *Tissot*, page 33.

50. *Convulsions.*

192. Use the *cold bath:*

193. Or, take a tea-spoonful of *valerian root* powdered, in a cup of water every evening:

194. Or, half a drachm of *misselto* powdered, every six hours, drinking after it a draught of strong infusion thereof.

51. *Convulsions in Children.*

195. Scrape *Piony roots* fresh digged.   Apply what you have scraped off to the soles of the feet.   It helps immediately. Tried.

52. *Convulsions in the Bowels of Children.*

196. Give a child a quarter old, a spoonful of the juice of *pellitory of the wall*, two or three times a day.   It goes through at once, but purges no more.   Use the syrup, if the juice cannot be had.

53. *Corns (to prevent.)*

197. Frequently wash the feet in *cold water.*

54. *Corns (to cure.)*

198. Apply fresh every morning the *yeast* of small beer, spread on a rag:

199. Or, after paring them close, apply bruised *ivy-leaves* daily, and in fifteen days they will drop out: tried.

200. Or, apply *chalk* powdered and mixt with water.   This also cures warts.

201. Some corns are cured by a *pitch plaister.*

202. All are greatly eased by steeping the feet in hot water wherein *oatmeal* is boiled.   This also helps dry and hot feet.

58

203. Rise early every morning:

204. Or, boil in a pint and a half of broth, half a handful of *mallow-leaves* chopt: strain this and drink it, before you eat any thing else.   Do this frequently, if needful:

205. Or, breakfast twice a week or oftener, on *water-gruel with currants:* tried.

206. Or, take the bigness of a large nutmeg of *cream of tartar* mixt with *honey*, as often as you need.

207. Or, take daily two hours before dinner a small tea-cupful of *stewed-prunes:*

208. Or, use for common drink, *water*, or *treacle-beer*, impregnated with *fixed air:*[1]

209. Or, live upon *bread*, made of *wheat-flour*, with all the bran in it.

210. Or, boil an ounce and a half of *tamarinds* in three pints of water to a quart.   In this strained, when cold, infuse all night two drachms of *sena*, and one drachm of *red rose-leaves*, drink a cup every morning.—See Dr. *Tissot.*

56. *A Cough.*

211. Every cough is a dry cough at first.   As long as it continues so, it may be cured by chewing immediately after you cough, the quantity of a pepper-corn of *Peruvian bark*.   Swallow your spittle as long as it is bitter, and then spit out the wood.   If you cough again, do this again.   It very seldom fails to cure any dry cough.   I earnestly desire every one who has any regard for his health to try this within twenty-four hours, after he first perceives a cough.

212. Or, drink a pint of *cold water* lying down in bed: tried.

213. Or, make a hole through a *lemon* and fill it with *honey*. Roast it, and catch the juice.   Take a tea-spoonful of this frequently: tried.

[1 Fixed air is Carbonic Acid Gas.   See No. 682.]

57. *An Asthmatic Cough.*

214. Take *Spanish liquorice* two ounces, *salt of tartar* half an ounce: boil the liquorice in three pints of water to a quart. Add the *salt* to it when it is blood-warm. Drink two spoonfuls of this every two hours. It seldom fails: tried.—I have known this cure an inveterate moist asthma.

58. *A Consumptive Cough.*

215. To stop it for a time, at lying down keep a little *stick liquorice* shaved like *horse-radish*, between the cheek and the gums. I believe this never fails.

59. *A Convulsive Cough.*

216. Eat preserved *walnuts.*

60. *An Inveterate Cough.*

217. Wash the head in *cold water* every morning:

218. Or, use the *cold bath:*—It seldom fails:

219. Or, peel and slice a large *turnip*, spread *coarse sugar* between the slices, and let it stand in a dish till all the juice drains down. Take a spoonful of this whenever you cough:

220. Or, take a spoonful of syrup of *horehound*, morning and evening: tried.

221. Or, take from ten to twenty drops of *Elixir of Vitriol* [see p. 42], in a glass of water twice or thrice a day. This is useful when the cough is attended with costiveness, or relaxation of the stomach and lungs.

61. *A Pleuritic Cough.*

222. Powder an ounce of *sperma-ceti* fine. Work it in a marble mortar with the yolk of a new-laid egg. Mix them in a pint of white wine, and take a small glass every three hours.

62. *A Tickling Cough.*

223. Drink *water* whitened with oatmeal four times a day:

224. Or, keep a piece of *barley-sugar*, or *sugar-candy* constantly in the mouth.

63. *Violent Coughing from a sharp and thin Rheum.*

225. Work into old *conserve of roses*, as much as you can of pure *frankincense* powdered as fine as possible. Take a bolus of this twice or thrice a day. It eases presently, and cures in two or three weeks:

226. Or, take half a grain of the inspissated milky juice of *sowthistle*, once or twice a day. It has the anodyne and antispasmodic properties of opium, without its narcotic effects. Or, it may be made into laudanum, in the same manner as opium is, and five or six drops taken on a lump of sugar, thrice a day.

The milky juice of all the sowthistles, dandelions, and lettuces, have nearly the same virtues.

227. Or, use *milk* diet as much as possible.

64. *The Cramp (to prevent.)*

228. Tie your garter smooth and tight under your knee at going to bed: It seldom fails.

229. Or, take half a pint of *tar-water*, morning and evening:

230. Or, be *electrified* through the part which uses to be affected. This generally prevents it for a month: sometimes for a twelvemonth.

231. Or to one ounce and a half of *spirits of turpentine*, add *flour of brimstone* and *sulphur vivum*, of each half an ounce; smell to it at night, three or four times:

232. Or, lay a roll of brimstone under your pillow.

65. *The Cramp (to cure.)*

233. Strongly put out your heel:

234. Or, chafe the part with *Hungary-water:*[1]

[1 A distilled water prepared from the tops of flowers of Rosemary or other aromatic substances—so called because prepared for a Queen of Hungary.]

235. Or, hold a roll of *brimstone* in your hand. I have frequently done this with success.

66. *A Cut.*

236. Keep it closed with your thumb a quarter of an hour. Then double a rag five or six times; dip it in cold water, and bind it on: tried.

237. Or, bind on *toasted cheese.* This will cure a deep cut.

238. Or pounded *grass.* Shake it off after twelve hours, and if need be, apply fresh.

67. *Deafness.*

239. Be *electrified* through the ear: Tried.

240. Or, use the *cold bath:*

241. Or, put a little *salt* into the ear:

242. Or, drop into it a tea-spoonful of *salt water:*

243. Or, three or four drops of *onion-juice* at lying down, and stop it with a little wool.

68. *Deafness from Wax.*

244. Syringe the ear with warm *water:*—Tried.

69. *Deafness with a Dry Ear.*

245. Mix *brandy* and *sweet oil:* dip black wool in this, and put it into the ear. When it grows dry, wash it well in brandy; dip it and put it in again.

70. *Deafness with a Head-ach and Buzzing in the Head.*

246. Peel a clove of *garlick:* dip it in *honey,* and put it into your ear at night with a little black wool. Lie with that ear uppermost. Do this, if need be, eight or ten nights. Tried.

71. *A settled Deafness.*

247. Take a red *onion,* pick out the core; fill up the place with oil of *roasted almonds.* Let it stand a night; then bruise

and strain it. Drop three or four drops into the ear, morning and evening, and stop it with black wool.

72. *Delivery.*

248. After *delivery* in child-birth the mother's milk is the only proper purge for the child. Let it begin to suck ten or twelve hours after the birth.

73. *A Diabetes.*†

249. Drink wine boiled with *ginger*, as much and as often as your strength will bear. Let your drink be milk and water. All milk meats are good.

250. Or, drink three or four times a day a quarter of a pint of *alum* posset, putting three drachms of *alum* to four pints of milk. It seldom fails to cure in eight or ten days. (Dr. MEAD.)

251. Or, infuse half an ounce of *cantharides* in a pint of *Elixir of Vitriol*. Give from fifteen to thirty drops in *Bristol*[1] *water*, twice or thrice a day.

74. *The Dropsy.*‡

252. Use the *cold bath* daily, after purging:

253. Or, rub the swelled parts with *salled* [salad] *oil* by a warm hand, at least an hour a day. This has done wonders in some cases.

254. Or, cover the whole belly with a large new sponge dipt in strong *lime-water*, and then squeezed out. This bound on often cures, even without any sensible evacuation of water.

255. Or, apply green *dock-leaves* to the joints and soles of the feet, changing them once a day.

* A *diabetes* is a frequent and large discharge of pale and sweetish urine, attended with a constant thirst, and a wasting of the whole body.

‡ A *dropsy* is a preternatural collection of water in the head, breast, belly, or all over the body. It is attended with a continual thirst. The part swelled pits if you press it with your fingers. The urine is pale and little.

[[1] A tepid water from springs at Clifton containing iron and sulphur. Formerly used for diseases of the lungs.]

256. Or, mix half an ounce of *amber* with a quart of wine *vinegar*. Heat a brick (only not red hot) and put it into a tub. Pour them upon it and hold the part swelled over the smoke. The water will come out incredibly, and the patient be cured: tried.

257. Or, eat a *crust of bread* every morning fasting: tried.

258. Or, take as much as lies on a six-pence of powdered *laurel-leaves*, every second or third day. It works both ways: tried.

259. Or, mix a pound of the coarsest *sugar* with a pint of juice of *Pellitory of the Wall*, bruised in a marble mortar. Boil it as long as any scum rises. When cool, bottle and cork it. If very bad, take three spoonfuls at night, and two in the morning. It seldom fails: tried.

260. Or, make tea of roots of *Dwarf Elder*. It works by urine. Every twelve or fourteen minutes, (that is, after every discharge) drink a tea-cup full.—I have known a dropsy cured by this in twelve hours time.

261. One was cured, by taking a drachm of *nitre* every morning in a little ale.

262. *Tar-water* drank twice a day has cured many; so has an infusion of *juniper berries* roasted, and made into a liquor like coffee:

263. Or three spoonfuls of the juice of *leeks*, or *elder-leaves*: tried.——This cures the windy dropsy.

264. Or, half a pint of decoction of *Butchers Broom* (inter-mixing purges twice or thrice a week.) The proper purge is ten grains of *jalap*, with six of powdered *ginger*. It may be increased or lessened according to the strength of the patient:

265. Or, of the decoction of the tops of *oak-boughs*. This cured an inveterate dropsy in fifteen days:

266. Or, take *sena*, *cream of tartar* and *jalap*, half an ounce of each. Mix them and take a drachm every morning in broth. It usually cures in twenty days. This is nearly

the same with Dr. *Ward's* powder. I suppose he took it from hence. He says it seldom fails, either in the watry or windy *dropsy*.

267. Or, be *electrified:* this cures dropsies supposed incurable.

268. ☞ *How amazingly little is yet known, even of the human body! Have not dropsical persons been continually advised to obstain from drink as much as possible? But how can we reconcile this with the following undeniable facts, published in the late* Medical Transactions?

Jane Roberts, aged twenty, was at length constrained to take her bed by a confirmed *ascites* and *anasarca*. In this desperate case, she drank as much as she would, first of *small beer*, and when that failed, of *thin milk*. After awhile her skin cracked in many places: and she continued drinking and leaking till she was quite well.

A middle-aged man in the West of *England*, drank every day five or six quarts of *cyder:* and without any other medicine, was totally cured in a few weeks time of a dropsy long supposed to be incurable.

A Farmer aged seventy, in a confirmed *ascites*, was given over for dead. Being desperate, he drank three quarts of *cold water*, every four and twenty hours. His whole food meantime was sea-biscuit, sometimes with a little butter. For sixteen days he seemed worse. Then he discharged for near a week a vast quantity of water, and was soon free from his disease, which never returned.

75. *Drowned.*

269. Rub the trunk of the body all over with *salt*. It frequently recovers them that seem dead.—See Extract from Dr. *Tissot*, page 150.

76. *The Ear-Ach.*

270. Rub the ear hard for a quarter of an hour. Tried.

271. Or, be *electrified:*

272. Or, put in a roasted *fig*, or *onion*, as hot as may be: tried.

273. Or, blow the *smoke of tobacco* strongly into it.

274. But if the ear-ach is caused by an inflammation of the uvula, it is cured in two or three hours, by receiving into the mouth the steam of bruised *hemp-seed*, boiled in water.

77. *Ear-Ach from Cold.*

275. Boil *rue*, or *rosemary*, or *garlick*, and let the steam go into the ear through a funnel.

78. *Ear-Ach from Heat.*

276. Apply cloths four times doubled and dipt in *cold water*, changing them when warm, for half an hour.

79. *Ear-Ach from Worms:*

277. Drop in *warm milk*, and it brings them out:

278. Or, juice of *wormwood*, which kills them.

80. *Noise in the Ears.*

279. Drop in juice of *onions*.

81. *Hard Wax in the Ear.*

280. Is best dissolved by *warm water*.

82. *Eyes bleared.*

281. Drop into them the juice of *crab-apples*.

83. *A Blood-shot Eye.*

282. Apply linen rags dipt in *cold water* for two or three hours:

283. Or blow in white *sugar-candy*, finely powdered:

284. Or, apply boiled *hyssop* as a poultice. This has a wonderful efficacy.

84. *A Bruise in the Eye.*

285. Apply as a plaister, *conserve of roses*.

85. *Clouds flying before the Eye.*

286. Take a drachm of powdered *betony* every morning:

287. Or, be *electrified*.

86. *Blindness.*

288. Is often cured by *cold bathing:*

289. Or, by *electrifying:* tried.   This has cured a *suffusion* of sixteen, and a *gutta serena*[1] of twenty-four years standing.

87. *Dull Sight.*

290. Drop in two or three drops of juice of *rotten apples* often.

88. *Films.*

291. Dry *Zibethum Occidentale*, i.e. *Stercus humanum*, slowly; powder it fine, and blow it into the eye twice or thrice a day;

292. Or, mix juice of *ground-ivy*, with a little *honey*, and two or three grains of *Bay-salt:*——drop it in, morning and evening.

293. Or, touch them cautiously every day with the *lunar caustic* [silver nitrate].

89. *Hot or Sharp Humours.*

294. Apply a few drops of double-refined *sugar*, melted in *brandy:*—tried.

295. Or, boil a handful of *Bramble-leaves* with a little *alum* in a quart of spring-water, to a pint.   Drop this frequently into the eye.   This likewise speedily cures cankers or any sores.

296. Or, lay a thin slice of *raw beef* on the nape of the neck: tried.

[1 *Gutta Serena* is Amaurosis, blindness, especially blindness occurring without apparent cause.]

297. Apply as a poultice, *boiled*, *roasted*, or *rotten apples* warm.

298. Or, *wormwood-tops* with the *yolk* of an *egg:* —This will hardly fail.

299. Or, beat up the *white* of an *egg* with two spoonfuls of *white rose-water* into a white froth. Apply this on a fine rag, changing it so that it may not grow dry, till the eye or eye-lid is well: tried.

300. Or, dissolve an ounce of fine *gum arabic* in two or three spoonfuls of spring-water; put a drop into the inner corner of the eye, from the point of a hair-pencil, four or five times a day. At the same time take as much *salt petre* as will lie upon a six-pence, dissolved in a glass of water, three or four times a day; abstaining from all strong liquids as much as possible, till cured.—White bread poultices, applied to the eyes in an inflamed state, frequently occasion total blindness.

After the inflammation is subsided, if weakness still remains, dip a finger in the white copperas eye-water, and rub round the eye, three or four times a day.——N.B. All acrid eye-waters and powders, put into the eyes when they are inflamed, horribly increase both the pain and inflammation.

91. *Lachrymal Fistula.**

301. Apply a poultice of fine leaves of *rue:*

302. Or, wash the eye morning and evening with a decoction of *Quince-leaves*.

92. *Pearl in the Eye.*

303. Apply a drop of juice of *Celandine* with a feather thrice a day:

304. Or, of *three leaved grass.* It commonly cures in seven days:

* This disorder in the inner corner of the eye, causes the tears to flow involuntarily. When it is confirmed, only a Surgeon can cure it.

305. Or, dissolve a little *sal ammonica* [sal ammoniac] in *rose-water*. Keep this three days in a *copper* vessel. Drop it twice a day into the eye.

306. Or, reduce separately, to the finest powder possible, an equal weight of *loaf-sugar, cream of tartar,* and *bole armoniac;* mix them together, and put a little into the eye, (without blowing it in,) three or four times a day.

93. *Sore Eyes.*

307. Drink *eyebright* tea, and wash the eyes with it.

94. *White Specks in the Eye.*

*308. Going to bed, put a little *ear-wax* on the speck. This has cured many.

95. *An Excellent Eye-Water.*[1]

309. Put half an ounce of *lapis calaminaris* powdered, into half a pint of *French white wine* and as much *white rose-water:* drop a drop or two into the corner of the eye. It cures soreness, weakness, and most diseases of the eye. I have known it cure total blindness.

96. *Another.*

310. Boil very lightly one spoonful of *white copperas* scraped, and three spoonfuls of *white salt* in three pints of *spring-water.* When cold, bottle it in large vials, without straining. Take up the vial softly, and put a drop or two in the eye morning and evening.

☞ *It answers the intention of almost all the preceding medicines: it takes away redness, or any soreness whatever: it cures pearls, rheums, and often blindness itself. But it makes the eye smart.*

97. *Another.*

311. Stamp and strain *ground-ivy, celandine,* and *daisies* an equal quantity: add a little *rose-water* and *loaf-sugar.* Drop a drop or two at a time into the eye, and it takes

[1 See *Journal of John Wesley* (Standard Edn), IV. 373.]

away all manner of inflammation, smarting, itching, spots, webs, or any other disorder whatsoever, yea, though the sight were almost gone.

98. *An* EYE-WATER, *which was used by Sir* Stephen Fox, *when he was* 60 *years of age, and could hardly see with the help of spectacles; but hereby in some time he recovered his sight, and could read the smallest print without spectacles, till above eighty.*

312. Take five ounces of rectified *spirits of wine*, dissolve it in one drachm of *camphire:* then add two small handfuls of dried *elder flowers*.   In 24 hours after it is infused, it is ready for use.   Take out a little in a tea-spoon; dip your finger in it, and bathe your forehead, over your eyes, and each temple with it, several times, morning and night, and twice more in the day constantly.   Mean time dip a soft rag in dead small beer, new milk warm, and dab each eye a dozen times gently, morning and evening.

If it is a watry humour, you may with your finger wet the eye-lids two or three times a-piece: but be sure to shut your eyes, or it makes them smart and burn excessively. If you have the tooth-ach or swelled face, rub it well on the part, and it will take away the pain.   It will cure any bruise also, if used immediately: tried.

It will cure any inflammation in the eyes.

99. *Weak Eyes.*

313. Wash the head daily with *cold-water:* tried.

100. *Fainting on letting Blood.*

314. Is prevented by taking before it some good broth:

315. Or by lying on the bed, during the operation.

101. *The falling Sickness*† [*Epilepsy*].

316. Be *electrified:* tried.

† In the *Falling Sickness*, the patient falls to the ground, either quite stiff, or convulsed all over, utterly senseless, gnashing his teeth, and foaming at the mouth.

317. Or, use the *cold bath* for a month daily:

318. Or, take a tea-spoonful of *Piony root* dried and grated fine, morning and evening for three months:

319. Or, half a spoonful of *Valerian-root* powdered.—It often cures in twice taking:

320. Or, half a pint of *tar-water*, morning and evening, for three months:

321. Or, a glass of juice of *Pellitory of the wall*, every morning:

322. Or, take five or six drops of *laudanum* fasting, for six or seven mornings.——This has cured many:

323. Or, use an entire *milk diet* for three months: it seldom fails.

324. In the fit, blow up the nose a little powdered *ginger:*

325. Or, leaves of *assarabacca* powdered.——

☞ This is the famous *Major's* snuff.

*326. One who is subject to the Falling Sickness, may prevent the fit if he feels it coming, by this simple experiment. Let him always carry with him a piece of metal as broad as he is able to hold between his teeth, when his jaws are stretched to the utmost. When he feels the fit approaching, let him immediately put this between his teeth, so as to keep his jaws at their utmost stretch. In about a minute this will bring him quite to himself, and prevent the fit for that time.

If one put this metal between the teeth of one that is in the fit, and force them open, till his jaws are at the utmost stretch, the fit will immediately go off, and the patient very soon recover.

102. *The Falling of the Fundament.*[1]

327. Apply a cloth covered thick with *brick-dust:*

328. Or, boil a handful of *red rose-leaves* in a quarter of a pint of *red wine;* dip a cloth in it, and apply it as hot as can be borne. Do this till all is used.

[1 Rectocele, a protrusion of part of the Rectum.]

103. *A Falling down of the Womb.*

329. May be cured in the manner last mentioned:

330. Or, wear a Pessary of cork, and take once or twice a day a tea-cupful of the decoction of *the bark*, with ten drops of *Elixir of Vitriol*. [No. 46.]

104. *Extreme Fat.*

331. Use a total *vegetable diet*. I know one who was entirely cured of this, by living a year thus: she breakfasted and supped on milk and water (with bread) and dined on turnips, carrots, or other roots, drinking water.

105. *A Fever.*

(In the beginning of any fever, if the stomach is uneasy, vomit; if the bowels, purge: if the pulse be hard, full or strong, bleed.)

332. Drink a pint or two of *cold water* lying down in bed: I never knew it do hurt:

333. Or, a large glass of *tar-water* warm, every hour:

334. Or, thin *water-gruel* sweetened with *honey* with one or two drachms of *nitre* in each quart.

335. ☞ The best of all julaps [juleps][1] in a fever is this: Toast a large thin slice of bread, without burning; put it hot into a pint of cold water; then set it on the fire till it is pretty hot. In a dry heat it may be given cold; in a moist heat, warm; the more largely the better: tried.

336. Or, for a change, use *pippin* or *wood-sorrel* tea: or, *pippin-whey:* or, *wood-sorrel whey.*

337. (To prevent catching any infectious fever, do not breathe near the face of the sick person, neither swallow your spittle whilst in the room. Infection seizes the stomach first.)

338. Or, stamp a handful of leaves of *woodbine;* put fair water to it, and use it cold as a clyster. It often cures in an hour.

[1 Sweetened drinks or cordials.]

339. Or, smear the wrists, five or six inches long with warm *treacle*, and cover it with brown paper.—See Dr. *Tissot*.

340. Or, apply *treacle* plaisters to the head and the soles of the feet, changing them every twelve hours:

341. Or, use Doctor *Boerhaave's* fever-powder, viz. Eight ounces of *nitre*, a quarter of an ounce of *camphire*, half a quarter of an ounce of *saffron*, and eight grains of *cochineal*. These are to be powdered, mixt together, and kept dry in a bottle. Ten grains taken on going to bed abate feverish heat, and procure rest. Ten grains are to be taken every three or four hours for a continued fever.

106. *A high Fever.*

342. Attended with a delirium and a vigilia, has been cured by plunging into *cold water;* which is a safe and sure remedy in the beginning of any fever.

343. Such a delirium is often cured by applying to the top of the head, a *treacle* plaister: tried.

107. *An intermitting Fever.*

344. Drink warm *lemonade* in the beginning of every fit: it cures in a few days: tried.

345. Or, take a tea-spoonful of *oil of sulphur* in a cup of *balm-tea*, once or twice a day.

108. *A Fever with pains in the Limbs.*

346. Take twenty drops of *spirits of hartshorn* in a cup of water twice or thrice in twenty-four hours:

347. Or, drink largely of *cinquefoil* tea.

109. *A Rash Fever.*

348. Drink every hour a spoonful of juice of *ground-ivy*. It often cures in twenty-four hours.—Use the decoction when you have not the juice.

349. Use the *cold bath* for two or three weeks, daily.

111. *A Worm Fever.*

350. Boil a handful of *rue* and *wormwood* in water; foment the belly with the decoction, and apply the boiled herbs as a poultice; repeat the application night and morning. This frequently brings away worms from children, who will take no internal medicine; and is likewise serviceable, if the fever be of the putrid kind.

112. *A Fistula.*

351. Wash *muscle-shells* clean; burn them to powder; sift them fine: mix them with *hogs-lard;* spread it on clean washleather, and apply it. This cured one that was thought to be at the point of death.—N.B. This cures the piles.

352. Or, grind an ounce of *Mercury Sublimate*, in a glass mortar, with a glass pestle, as fine as possible. Put it into a glass bottle, and pour on it two quarts of pure spring-water. Cork it close, and for six days shake it well every hour. Then let it settle for twenty-four hours. Pour it off clear; filter in a glass funnel; and keep it for use close stopt. Put half a spoonful of this water in a phial, and add two spoonfuls of pure spring-water: shake them well together, and drink it fasting. It works both by vomit and by stool, but very safely. Keep yourself very warm, and walk as much as you can. The first time neither eat nor drink till two hours after it has done working. Take this every other day. In forty days this will also cure any *cancer*, any *old sore*, or *King's Evil*, broken or unbroken.—After the first or second vomit, you may use *water-gruel*, as in other vomits.

☞ *Very weak persons should not use this. But I have known it used safely and successfully.*

353. Or, have a vessel so contrived, that you may sit with the part in *cold water*, a quarter of an hour every morning. I have known a gentleman of seventy cured thereby.

354. Or, put a large stone of *unslacked lime* into four quarts of water, let it stand one night; take four ounces of *roche-alum* and four ounces of *white-copperas*, calcine them to dryness, then powder them as fine as possible: take three pints of the above water, and put the powder into it, and boil it for half an hour, then let it cool, and bottle it for use. Let the fistula be syringed with this often, a little warm; and make a tent to fit the place and dip in the water, and apply it twice a day. Cover it over with a plaister of diaculum.

This water will destroy the callosity of the edges of the fistula, which otherwise would prevent its healing, and if managed as above, will heal it up at the same time.

113. *To destroy Fleas and Bugs.*

355. Cover the floor of the room with leaves of *alder*, gathered while the dew hangs upon them: adhering to these, they are killed thereby.

356. Or, powder *stavesacre*, and sprinkle it on the body, or on the bed.

114. *Flegm.*

357. To prevent or cure, take a spoonful of *warm water*, the first thing in the morning.

115. *Flooding (in Lying-in.)*

358. Cover the body with cloths dipt in *vinegar* and *water*, changing them as they grow warm. Drink cooling, acid liquors.

This is a complaint which is never to be thought little of. Sometimes a violent flooding comes on before delivery; and the only way to save both the mother and child, is to deliver the woman immediately; which being done, the flooding will generally cease. Sometimes a slight flooding comes on some weeks before labour; and here, if the patient be kept cool, her diet light, and small doses of *nitre* often repeated, (an ounce divided into thirty parts, and one given every four hours,) she will frequently go her full time and do well: but if it should become excessive, delivery should be effected as soon as may be.

If a flooding should come on after delivery, the patient should be laid with her head low, kept cool, and be in all respects treated, as for an excessive flux of the *menses*. Linen cloths, which have been wrung out of vinegar and water, should be applied to the belly, the loins, and the thighs. These must be changed as they grow dry; and may be discontinued as soon as the flooding abates. Sometimes the following mixture will do great things, viz. *Pennyroyal-water*, simple *cinnamon-water*, and *syrup of poppies*, of each two ounces; *acid Elixir of Vitriol* one drachm. Mix, and take two table-spoonfuls every hour. But large doses of *nitre* given often (a scruple every hour,) is generally the most efficacious. But when all other things seem to have no effect, *cold water* dashed upon the patient's belly, will stop the flooding immediately.

116. *A Flux.*

359. Receive the smoke of *turpentine* cast on burning coals. This cures also the *bloody-flux*, and the *falling of the fundament*.

360. Or, put a large *brown toast* into three quarts of *water*, with a drachm of *cochineal* powdered, and a drachm of *salt of wormwood*. Drink it all in as short a time as you conveniently can.

☞ This rarely fails to cure all *fluxes, cholera morbus*, yea, and *inflammation of the bowels:* tried.

361. Or, take a spoonful of *Plantane-seed* bruised, morning and evening, till it stops:

362. Or, ten grains of *ipecacuanha*, three mornings successively. It is likewise excellent as a sudorific.

363. Or, boil four ounces of rasped *logwood*, or fresh *logwood chips*, in three quarts of water to two: strain it, and drink a quarter of a pint, sweetened with loaf-sugar, warm, twice a day. It both binds and heals: or, take a small tea-cupful of it every hour:

364. Or, boil the fat of a *breast of mutton* in a quart of water for an hour. Drink the broth as soon as you can conveniently. This will cure the most inveterate flux: tried.——See extract from Dr. *Tissot*, page 124.

117. *A Bloody Flux.*

365. Apply a suppository of linen dipt in *Aqua Vitæ* [Brandy].

366. Or, drink *cold water*, as largely as possible, taking nothing else till the flux stops:

367. Or, take a large *apple*, and at the top pick out all the core, and fill up the place with a piece of *honey-comb;* (the honey being strained out,) roast the apple in embers, and eat it, and this will stop the flux immediately:

368. Or, grated *rhubarb*, as much as lies on a shilling, with half as much of grated *nutmeg*, in a glass of *white wine*, at lying down every other night; tried.

369. Or, take four drops of *laudanum*, and apply to the belly a poultice of *wormwood* and *red roses* boiled in *milk*.

370. In a *Dysentery*, the worst of all fluxes, feed on *rice, saloup, sago*, and sometimes *beef-tea;* but no flesh.

371. To stop it, take a spoonful of *suet* melted over a slow fire. Do not let blood.

372. ☞ A person was cured in one day, by feeding on *rice-milk*, and sitting a quarter of an hour in a shallow tub, having in it warm *water* three inches deep.——See Extract from Dr. *Tissot*, page 125.

118. *To prevent (or stop a beginning) Gangrene.*

373. Foment continually with *vinegar*, in which *dross of iron* (either *sparks* or *clinkers*) has been boiled.

374. "Dissolve two drachms of *Venice-treacle* in a glass of *mountain* [*mountain wine*]. After drinking it, go to bed. You will be easier in two hours, and well in sixteen." (Dr. *Dover*.)

*375. Or, boil a pugil § of *tansey* in a quarter of a pint of *mountain*. Drink it in bed. I believe this never fails.

*376. To prevent its return, dissolve half an ounce of *gum guaiacum*, in two ounces of *sal volatile*. Take a tea-spoonful of this every morning in a glass of spring-water.

☞ *This helps any sharp pain in the stomach.*—Dr. *Boerhaave.*

N.B. I knew a gentleman who was cured many times by a large draught of *cold water.*

120. *The Gout in the Foot or Hand.*

377. Apply a raw lean *beef-steak.* Change it once in twelve hours, till cured. Tried.

121. *The Gout in any Limb.*†

*378. Rub the part with warm *treacle*, and then bind on a flannel smeared therewith. Repeat this, if need be, once in twelve hours.

☞ This has cured an inveterate gout in thirty-six hours.

379. Or, drink a pint of strong infusion of *elder-buds* dry or green, morning and evening. This has cured inveterate gouts.

380. Or at six in the evening, undress and wrap yourself up in blankets. Then put your legs up to the knees in water, as hot as you can bear it. As it cools, let hot

---

§ A *Pugil* is as much as you can take up between your thumb and two fore-fingers.

† Regard not them who say, The gout *ought not* to be cured. They mean, It *cannot.* I know it cannot by *their regular prescriptions.* But I have known it cured in many cases, without any ill effects following. I have cured myself several times.

water be poured in, so as to keep you in a strong sweat till ten. Then go into a bed well warmed and sweat till morning.——I have known this cure an inveterate gout, in a person above sixty, who lived eleven years after.—— The very matter of the Gout is frequently destroyed by a steady use of *Mynsicht's Elixir of Vitriol.*

122. *The Gravel.*

381. Eat largely of *Spinach:*

382. Or, drink largely of *warm water* sweetened with *honey:*

383. Or, of *pellitory of the wall* tea, so sweetened:

384. Or, infuse an ounce of *wild parsley-seeds* in a pint of *white wine* for twelve days. Drink a glass of it fasting, three months. To prevent its return, breakfast for three months on *agrimony* tea. It entirely cured me twenty years ago, nor have I had the least symptom of it since.

123. *The Green Sickness.*

385. Take an ounce of *quicksilver* every morning.

386. Or, a cup of decoction of *lignum guaiacum,* (commonly called *lignum vitæ,*) morning and evening.

387. Or, grind together into a fine powder three ounces of the finest *steel-filings,* and two ounces of *red sugar-candy.* Take from a scruple to half a drachm every morning. *I.* ——See Dr. *Tissot.*

124. *To kill Animalcula that cause the Gums to waste away from the teeth.*

388. Gargle thrice a day with *salt* and *water.*

125. *To make Hair grow.*

389. Wash it every night with a strong decoction of *rosemary.* Dry it with flannel: tried.

390. Rub the head for a quarter of an hour: tried.

391. Or, be *electrified:* tried.

392. Or, apply to each temple the thin yellow rind of a *lemon,* newly pared off.

393. Or, pour upon the palm of the hand a little *brandy,* and some zest* of *lemon,* and hold it to the forehead: or, a little ether:

394. Or, if you have catched cold, boil a handful of *rosemary* in a quart of water. Put this in a mug, and hold your head (covered with a napkin) over the steam, as hot as you can bear. Repeat this till the pain ceases: tried.

395. Or, snuff up the nose *camphorated spirits of lavender:*

396. Or, a little juice of *horse radish.*

127. *A Chronical Head-Ach.*

397. Keep your feet in *warm water,* a quarter of an hour before you go to bed, for two or three weeks: tried.

398. Or, wear tender *Hemlock-leaves* under the feet, changing them daily:

399. Or, order a tea-kettle of *cold water* to be poured on your head, every morning in a slender stream:

400. Or, take a large tea-cupful of *Cardus* [*Carduus*] tea, without sugar, fasting, for six or seven mornings: tried.

128. *Head-Ach from Heat.*

401. Apply to the forehead cloths dipt in *cold water* for an hour: tried.

129. *A Nervous Head-Ach.*

402. Dry and powder an ounce of *marjoram* and half an ounce of *assarabacca;* mix them and take them as snuff, keeping the ears and throat warm. This is of great use even in a

* *Zest* is the juice of the *peel* squeezed out.

cancer: but it will suffice to take a small pinch every other night, lying down in bed.

130. *A violent Head-Ach.*

403. Take of *white wine vinegar* and *water*, each three spoonfuls; with half a spoonful of *Hungary-water*. Apply this twice a day to the eye-lids and temples.

131. *Hemicrania.*§

404. Use *cold bathing:*

405. Or, apply to that part of the head shaved, a plaister, that will stick, with a hole cut in the middle of it as big as a half-penny: place over that hole leaves of *ranunculus*, bruised and very moist.   It is a gentle blister.

132. *Stoppage in the Head.*

406. Snuff up juice of *primrose*, keeping the head warm.

133. *The Heart-Burning.**

407. Drink a pint of *cold water:* tried.

438 [408]. Or, drink slowly decoction of *camomile flowers:*

409. Or, eat four or five *oysters:*

410. Or, chew five or six *pepper-corns* a little; then swallow them:

411. Or, chew *fennel* or *parsley*, and swallow your spittle.— Sometimes a *vomit* is needful.

412. Or, a piece of *Spanish-liquorice.*

134. *The Hiccup, (to prevent.)*

413. Infuse a scruple of *musk* in a quart of *mountain-wine*, and take a small glass every morning.

§ This is a *head-ach* which affects but one side of the head.
* A sharp gnawing pain in the orifice of the stomach.

414. Swallow a mouthful of *water*, stopping the mouth and ears: tried.

415. Or, take any thing that makes you sneeze:

416. Or, two or three preserved *damsons:*

417. Or, three drops of *oil of cinnamon*, on a lump of *sugar:* tried.

418. Or, ten drops of chymical *oil of amber* dropt on *sugar*, and then mixed with a little water.

135. *Hoarseness.*

*419. Rub the soles of the feet before the fire, with *garlick* and *lard* well beaten together, over night. The hoarseness will be gone the next morning: tried.

420. Or take a pint of *cold water* lying down:

421. Or, swallow slowly the juice of *radishes:*

422. Or, half a pint of *mustard-whey*, lying down:

423. Or, a tea-spoonful of *conserve of roses*, every night: tried.

424. Or, dry *nettle-roots* in an oven. Then powder them finely, and mix with an equal quantity of *treacle*. Take a tea-spoonful of this twice a day.

425. Or, boil a large handful of *wheat-bran* in a quart of water; strain, and sweeten it with *honey*. Sup of it frequently.

136. *Hypochondriac and Hysteric Disorders.*

426. Use *cold bathing:*

427. Or, take an ounce of *quicksilver* every morning, and ten drops of *Elixir of Vitriol* in the afternoon, in a glass of *cold water.*

137. *The Jaundice.*

428. Wear leaves of *celandine* upon and under the *feet:*

429. Or, take a small pill of *castile-soap* every morning, for eight or ten days: tried.

430. Or, beat the *white of an egg* thin: take it morning and evening in a glass of water: *I.*

431. Or half a pint of strong decoction of *nettles:* or, of *Burdock-leaves,* morning and evening.

432. Or, boil three ounces of *Burdock-root,* in two quarts of water to three pints. Drink a tea-cupful of this every morning.

138. *Jaundice in Children.*

433. Take half an ounce of fine *rhubarb,* powdered. Mix with it thoroughly, by long beating, two handfuls of good well-cleansed *currants.* Of this give a tea-spoonful every morning.

139. *The Iliac [Ileac] Passion.**[1]

434. Apply warm flannels soaked in *spirits of wine:*

435. Or hold a *live puppy* constantly on the belly. (Dr. *Sydenham.*)

436. Or, immerge up to the breast in a *warm bath:*

437. Or, take, ounce by ounce, a pound, or a pound and a half of *quicksilver.*—(See Dr. *Tissot,* page 120.)

Inflammations in general are more certainly abated by smart *purging* than by bleeding.

140. *An Imposthume [an Abscess].*

438. Put the white of two *leeks* in a wet cloth, and so roast them in ashes, but not too much. Stamp them in a mortar with a little *hogs-grease.* Spread it thick, plaister-wise, and apply it, changing it every hour, till all the matter be come out, which will be in three times. *I.*

* In this violent kind of *Cholic* the excrements are supposed to be thrown up by the mouth in vomiting.

[1 *Ilium* refers to the bone, *Ileum* refers to the bowel. Ileac Passion is obstruction of the bowel.]

141. *The Itch [Scabies]*.‡

439. Wash the parts affected, with *strong rum:* tried.

440. Or, anoint them with *black soap;* but wash it off soon.

*441. Or, steep a shirt half an hour in a quart of water, mixed with half an ounce of powdered *brimstone*. Dry it slowly, and wear it five or six days. Sometimes it needs repeating: tried.

442. Or, mix powder of *white hellebore* with *cream* for three days. Anoint the joints three mornings and evenings.— It seldom fails.

443. Or, beat together the juice of two or three *lemons*, with the same quantity of *oil of roses*. Anoint the parts affected. It cures in two or three times using.

142. *The King's Evil [Scrofula]*.*

444. Take as much *cream of tartar* as lies on a sixpence, every morning and evening:

445. Or, drink for six weeks half a pint of a strong decoction of *devil's bit:* tried.

*446. Or, use the diet-drink, as in the article *scorbutic sores* [ART. 198]. I have known this cure one whose breast was as full of holes as a honey-comb.

447. Or, set a quart of *honey* by the fire to melt. When it is cold, strew into it a pound and a half of *quick-lime* beat very fine, and sifted through a hair-sieve. Stir this about, till it boil up of itself into a hard lump. Beat it when cold, very fine, and sift it as before. Take of this as much as lies on a shilling in a glass of water, every morning, an hour before breakfast, at four in the afternoon, and at going to bed:

‡ This distemper is nothing but a kind of very small lice, which burrow under the skin. Therefore inward medicines are absolutely needless.——Is it possible any Physician should be ignorant of this?

* It commonly appears first, by the thickness of the lips; or a stubborn humour in the eyes; then come hard swellings in the neck chiefly; then running sores.

448. Or, make a leaf of dried *burdock* into a pint of tea. Take half a pint twice a day, for four months. I have known this cure hundreds.

449. The best purge for the King's Evil is *Tincture of jalap*, which is made thus:—jalap in powder, three ounces; Geneva, or proof spirits, one pint. Let them infuse seven days. A tea-spoonful or two is sufficient for a child ten years old, in a morning fasting; and repeated once a week, so as to keep the stomach and bowels clean, will frequently cure the King's Evil. But all violent purges, when repeated too often, are pernicious.

143. *Lameness, from a fixed Contraction of the Parts.*

450. Beat the *yolk* of a new-laid egg very thin, and by a spoonful at a time, add and beat up with it three ounces of water. Rub this gently into the parts for a few minutes, three or four times a day.

144. *Legs inflamed.*

*451. Apply *Fuller's-earth* spread on brown paper. It seldom fails:

452. Or, bruised *turnips*.

145. *Legs Sore and Running.*

453. Wash them in *brandy*, and apply *elder-leaves*, changing them twice a day. This will dry up all the sores, though the legs were like a honeycomb: tried.

454. Or, poultice them with *rotten apples:* tried. But take also three or four purges.

146. *Leprosy.**

455. Use the *cold-bath:*

456. Or, wash in the sea, often and long:

* In this disease, the skin in many parts is covered with rough, whitish, scaly pustules; and if these are rubbed off, with a kind of scaly scurf.

457. Or, mix well an ounce of *pomatum*, a drachm of powdered *brimstone*, and half an ounce of *sal prunellæ;* and anoint the parts so long as there is need:

458. Or, add a pint of juice of *houseleek*, and half a pint of *verjuice*, to a pint and a half of *whey*. Drink this in twenty-four hours:———It often cures the quinsey, and white swellings on the joints:

459. Or, drink half a pint of *cellery whey*, morning and evening. This has cured in a most desperate case:

460. Or drink for a month, a decoction of *burdock-leaves*, morning and evening: tried.

147. *Lethargy.*

461. Snuff strong *vinegar* up the nose:

462. Or, take half a pint of decoction of *water-cresses*, morning and evening.

148. *Lice, (to kill.)*

463. Sprinkle *Spanish snuff*, over the head:

464. Or, wash it with a decoction of *amaranth*.

149. *For one seemingly killed with Lightning, a Damp, or suffocated.*

465. Plunge him immediately into *cold water:*

466. Or, blow strongly with bellows down his throat. This may recover a person seemingly drowned. It is still better, if a strong man blows into his mouth.

150. *Lues Venerea.*

467. Take an ounce of *quicksilver* every morning, and a spoonful of *aqua sulphurata* in a glass of *water*, at five in the afternoon. I have known a person cured by this, when supposed to be at the point of death, who had been infected by a foul nurse, before she was a year old.

☞ I insert this for the sake of such innocent sufferers.

468. Give decotion of *agrimony* four times a day:

469. Or, rub the head several times a day with *vinegar*, in which *ground-ivy leaves* have been infused:

470. Or, take daily an ounce of *distilled vinegar:*

471. Or, boil juice of *ground-ivy* with *sweet oil* and *white wine* into an ointment. Shave the head, anoint it therewith, and chafe it in warm every other day for three weeks. Bruise also the leaves and bind them on the head, and give three spoonfuls of the juice warm every morning.

☞ This generally cures melancholy.

The juice alone, taken twice a day, will cure.

472. Or, *electrify:* tried.

152. *Raging Madness.*§

473. Apply to the head, cloths dipt in *cold water:*

474. Or, set the patient with his head under a great *water-fall,* as long as his strength will bear: or, pour water on his head out of a tea-kettle:

475. Or, let him eat nothing but *apples* for a month:

476. Or, nothing but *bread* and *milk:* tried.

153. *The Bite of a Mad Dog.*

477. Plunge into *cold water* daily for twenty days, and keep as long under it as possible.—This has cured, even after the *hydrophobia* was begun.‖

478. Or, mix ashes of *trefoil* with *hog's-lard*, and anoint the part as soon as possible. Repeat it twice or thrice at six hours distance.

§ It is a sure rule, that all madmen are cowards, and may be conquered by binding only, without beating. (Dr. MEAD.) He also observes, that blistering the head does more harm than good. Keep the head close shaved, and frequently wash it with *vinegar*.

‖ If this is really a nervous disorder, what wonder if it should be cured by *cold bathing?*

☞ This has cured many: and particularly a dog bit on the nose by a mad dog.

479. Or, mix a pound of *salt*, with a quart of water. Squeeze, bathe, and wash the wound with this for an hour. Then bind some salt upon it for twelve hours.

N.B. *The Author of this receipt was bit six times by mad dogs, and always cured himself by this means.*

480. Or, mix powdered *liver-wort*, four drachms: *black pepper*, two drachms. Divide this into four parts, and take one in *warm milk* for four mornings fasting. Dr. *Mead* affirms he never knew this fail:—But it has sometimes failed.

481. Or, take two or three spoonfuls of the juice of *ribwort*, morning and evening, as soon as possible after the bite. Repeat this for two or three changes of the moon. It has not been known to fail.

154. *The Measles.*‡

☞ Immediately consult an honest Physician.

482. Drink only thin *water-gruel*, or *milk* and *water*, the more the better; or *toast* and *water*.

483. If the cough be very troublesome, take frequently a spoonful of *barley-water* sweetened with *oil of sweet almonds* newly drawn, mixed with syrup of *maiden-hair*.

484. After the measles, take three or four purges, and for some weeks take care of catching cold; use light diet, and drink *barley-water*, instead of malt-drink.—See Extract from Dr. *Tissot*, p. 82.

155. *Menses obstructed.*

485. Be *electrified:* tried.

486. Or, take half a pint of strong decoction of *penny-royal*, every night at going to bed:

‡ This distemper is always preceded by a violent cough, often fourteen days before the red spots come out.

487. Or, boil five large heads of *hemp*, in a pint of water to half. Strain it and drink it at going to bed, two or three nights. It seldom fails: tried.

488. Or, take from eight to twelve grains of *calomel*, in a pill, for two or three nights, taking care not to catch cold. It vomits and purges; tried.

489. Or, pour twelve ounces of rectified spirits of wine on four ounces of roots of *black hellebore*, and let it stand in a warm place twenty-four hours. Pour it off, and take from thirty to forty drops in any liquid, fasting:

It is good likewise in the Green Sickness; in all hypochondriacal cases, and in obstinate madness.

490. Or, burn a little *Sulphur of Antimony* on a chafing-dish of coals, and receive the smoke by a funnel. In a few minutes it will take effect.

☞ *Let any of these medicines be used at the* regular *time as near as can be judged.*—See Dr. TISSOT.

156. *Menses Nimii.*

491. Drink nothing but *cold water*, with a spoonful of fine *flour* stirred in it. At that time drink a glass of the *coldest water* you can get, and apply a thick cloth dipt in cold water:

492. Or, put the feet into *cold water:*

493. Or, apply a sponge dipt in *red wine* and *vinegar:*

494. Or, *bleed* in the arm. Stop the orifice often with the finger, and then let it bleed again:

495. Or, boil four or five leaves of the *red hollyhock* in a pint of milk, with a small quantity of sugar. Drink this in the morning: if the person can afford it, she may add a tea-spoonful of *Balm of Gilead*.[1]—This does not often fail:

*496. Or, reduce to a fine powder half an ounce of *alum*, with a quarter of an ounce of *dragon's blood*.[2] In a violent case, take a quarter of a drachm every half hour. It

[[1] Dragon's Blood. [2] A red resin from various tropical trees.]

scarce ever fails to stop the flux, before half an ounce is taken.

This also cures the *whites*.

157. *To resolve coagulated Milk.*

497. Cover the woman with a table-cloth, and hold a pan of *hot water* just under her breast; then stroke it three or four minutes. Do this twice a day, till it is cured.

158. *To increase Milk.*

498. Drink a pint of *water* going to bed:

499. Or, drink largely of *pottage* made with *lentils*.

159. *To make Milk agree with the Stomach.*

500. If it lie heavy, put a little *salt* in it; if it curdle, *sugar*. For bilious persons mix it with water.

160. *A Mortification,* (*to stop.*)

501. Apply a poultice of *flour*, *honey*, and *water*, with a little *yeast*.

161. *Nervous Disorders.*

502. When the nerves perform their office too languidly, a GOOD AIR is the first requisite. The patient also should rise early, and as soon as the dew is off the ground, walk: let his breakfast be *Mother of Thyme* tea, gathered in *June*, using half as much as we do of common tea. When the nerves are too sensible, let the person breathe a proper air. Let him eat veal, chickens, or mutton. Vegetables should be eat sparingly; the most innocent is the French bean; and the best root, the turnip. Wine should be avoided carefully: so should all sauces. Sometimes he may breakfast upon a quarter of an ounce of the powder of *Valerian root* infused in hot water, to which he may add cream and sugar. Tea is not proper. When

the person finds an uncommon oppression, let him take a large spoonful of the tincture of *Valerian root*.

☞ *This* tincture *should be made thus:——Cut to pieces six ounces of wild* Valerian-root, *gathered in* June, *and fresh dried. Bruise it by a few strokes in a mortar, that the pieces may be split, but it should not be beat into powder: put this into a quart of strong white wine: cork the bottle and let it stand three weeks, shaking it every day; then press it out and filter the tincture through paper.*

N.B. The true, wild *Valerian* has no bad smell: if it has, cats have urined upon it, which they will do, if they can come at it.

503. But I am firmly persuaded, there is no remedy in nature, for nervous disorders of every kind, comparable to the proper and constant use of the *electrical machine*.

162. *Nettle Rash.*§

504. Rub the parts strongly with *parsley*. Internals profit nothing.

163. *Old Age.*

505. Take *tar-water* morning and evening: tried.

506. Or, decoction of *nettles:* either of these will probably renew their strength for some years:

507. Or, be *electrified* daily:

508. Or, chew *cinnamon* daily, and swallow your spittle.

164. *An old stubborn Pain in the Back.*

509. Steep root of *water fern* in water, till the water become thick and clammy. Then rub the parts therewith morning and evening:

§ A slight fever, (which sometimes lasts for weeks) attended with itching and smarting, and an eruption all over the body, just like that occasioned by nettles. In *Georgia*, we called it, *The prickly heat.*

510. Or, apply a plaister, and take daily Balsam of *Capivi*.—
Or, apply *garlick* and *hog's lard* to the feet, as ART. 418.
[ART. 135, No. 419]. Tried.

165. *The Palsy.*‡

511. Be *electrified* daily for three months, from the places
wherein the nerves spring, which are brought to the
paralytic part.—If the parts beneath the head are affected,
the fault is in the spinal marrow. If half the body, half
the marrow is touched.

☞ A *palsy* may be cured in spring or summer, but rarely in
winter.

512. Or, use the *cold bath*, if you are under fifty, rubbing and
sweating after it:

513. Or, shred white *onions*, and bake them gently in an
earthen pot, till they are soft; spread a thick plaister of
this, and apply it to the benumbed part, all over the side,
if need be.——I have known this cure a person 75 years
old.

514. Or, take *tar-water* morning and evening.

515. Or, boil *white* and *red sage*, a handful of each in a quart
of *white wine*. Strain and bottle it. Take a small glass
morning and evening.

☞ *This helps all nervous disorders.*

516. Or, take a tea-spoonful of powdered *sage* lying down in
bed.

166. *Palsy of the Hands.*

517. Wash them often in decoction of *sage*, as hot as you can
bear:

518. Or, boil a handful of *elder-leaves*, or two or three spoonfuls of *mustard-seed* in a quart of water. Wash as often
in this, as hot as may be.

‡ A *palsy* is the loss of motion or feeling, or both, in any particular part
of the body.

167. *Palsy of the Mouth.*

519. After purging well, chew *mustard-seed* often:

520. Or, gargle with juice of *wood-sage.*

168. *Palsy from working with white Lead or Verdigrease.*

521. Use *warm baths* and a milk diet.

169. *The Palpitation, or beating of the Heart.*

522. Drink a pint of *cold water:*

523. Or, apply outwardly a rag dipt in *vinegar:*

524. Or, be *electrified:* tried.

525. Or, take a decoction of *Mother's-wort*[1] every night.

170. *The Piles (to prevent.)*

526. Wash the parts daily with *cold water.*

171. *The Piles (to cure.)*

527. Apply warm *treacle:*

528. Or, a *tobacco-leaf* steeped in water twenty-four hours:

529. Or, a poultice of boiled *brook-lime.*   It seldom fails:

530. Or, a bruised *onion* skinned; or roasted in ashes.   It perfectly cures the dry piles:

531. Or, *varnish.*   It perfectly cures both the blind and bleeding piles: tried.

532. Or, fumigate with *vinegar*, wherein red hot *flints* have been quenched.   This softens even schirrhous tumours.

172. *The inward Piles.*

533. Swallow a pill of *pitch*, fasting.   One pill usually cures the bleeding piles:

534. Or, eat a large *leek*, boiled:

535. Or, take twice a day, as much as lies on a shilling, of the *thin skin of walnuts*, powdered.

[1 Motherwort, *Leonurus Cardiaca,* a pale, roseate, mint-like flower formerly given in chest complaints.]

173. *Violent Bleeding Piles.*

536. Lightly boil *juice of nettles*, with a little *sugar:* take two
ounces.   It seldom needs repeating.

174. *The Plague (to prevent.)*

537. Eat *marigold flowers* daily, as a sallad, with *oil* and
vinegar:

538. Or infuse *rue, sage, mint, rosemary, worm-wood,* of each
a handful, into two quarts of the sharpest *vinegar,* over
warm embers for eight days.   Then strain it through a
flannel, and add half an ounce of *camphire,* dissolved in
three ounces of rectified *Spirits of wine.*   With this
wash the loins, face, and mouth, and snuff a little up the
nose when you go abroad.   Smell to a sponge dipt therein, when you approach infected persons or places.

N.B. This is the famous *Marseilles* vinegar.

175. *The Plague (to cure.)*

539. *Cold water* alone, drank largely, has cured it:

540. Or, an ounce or two of the juice of *marigolds:*

541. Or, after bleeding fifty or sixty ounces, drink very largely
of water sharpened with Spirit of *vitriol:*

542. Or, a draught of *brine* as soon as seized: sweat in bed;
take no other drink for some hours:

Or, use *lemon-juice* largely in every thing.

176. *The Pleurisy.**[1]

543. Take half a drachm of *soot:*

544. Or, take out the core of an apple; fill it with white
frankincense; stop it close with the piece you cut out, and
roast it in ashes.   Mash and eat it.   *I.*

545. Or, a glass of *tar-water* warm, every half hour:

---

* A *Pleurisy* is a fever attended with a violent pain in the side and a pulse
remarkably hard.

[[1] See *Journal of John Wesley* (Standard Edn), IV. 109, 156, 196.]

546. Or, a decoction of *nettles;* and apply the boiled herb hot, as a poultice. I never knew it fail.

547. Or, a plaister of *flour of brimstone* and *white of an egg:* tried.——(See Dr. *Tissot,* page 38.) This seldom fails:

548. In disorders of this kind, Dr. *Huxham* advises, "Sip almost continually thin *whey, barley-water,* or *hyssop-tea,* sharpened with *lemon-juice* or *vinegar* and *water.* If the spitting stop suddenly, take a little vomit. Likewise camphorated *vinegar,* with syrup of elder or rasberries, is good. To appease the cough, take often, a little at a time, of roasted apples, of strawberries, rasberries, or currants.

177. *To one Poisoned.*

549. Give one or two grains of *distilled verdigrease:* it vomits in an instant.

550. Let one poisoned by *arsenic* dissolve a quarter of an ounce of *salt of tartar* in a pint of water, and drink every quarter of an hour as much as he can, till he is well.

551. Let one poisoned by *opium* take thirty drops of *Elixir of Vitriol* in cold water, every quarter of an hour, till the drowsiness or wildness ceases:

552. Or, a spoonful of *lemon-juice.*

553. Let one poisoned with *mercury sublimate* dissolve an ounce of *salt of tartar* in a gallon of water, and drink largely of it. ☞ This will entirely destroy the force of the poison, if it be used soon.

554. Nothing cures the *African* poison, but a decoction of the roots of the *sensitive plant.*

178. *Polypus in the Nose.*

555. Powder a lump of *alum,* and snuff it up frequently. Then dissolve powdered *alum* in *brandy:* dip lint therein, and apply it at going to bed.

179. *A Prick or Cut that festers.*

556. Apply *turpentine.*

180. *Ptyalism.†*

557. A very violent and stubborn disorder of this kind was cured by *chewing* perpetually a little *dry bread*, and swallowing it with the spittle.

181. *An easy Purge.*

558. Drink a pint of warmish *water* fasting, walking after it:

559. Or, a *soft egg* with a tea-spoonful of *salt:*

560. Or, infuse from half a drachm, to two drachms of *Damask rose leaves* dried, in half a pint of warm water, for twelve hours, and take it.

561. Or, infuse three drachms of *sena*, and a scruple of *salt of tartar*, in half a pint of river water for twelve hours. Then strain and take it in the morning.

562. *Wild-ash* is a plant of the very same nature with *sena*. Its leaves taken in the same quantity purge full as well, and do not gripe as *sena* does.   It is therefore preferable to that which is brought from *Turkey* or *Italy*.

☞ The *Wild-ash* is called in the North of England, *round-tree, quicken, quick-beam*, or *Wiggan-tree*. The leaves should be gathered, when the tree is in flower.

182. *A stronger Purge.*

563. Drink half a pint of strong decoction of *dock-root:*

564. Or, two drachms of the powdered root of *Monks rhubarb*, with a scruple of *ginger*.

183. *The Quinsy.**

565. Apply a large white-bread toast, half an inch thick, dipt in *brandy*, to the crown of the head, till it dries:

566. Or, swallow slowly *white rose-water*, mixed with syrup of *mulberries:* tried.

567. Or, juice or jelly of *black currants*, or decoction of the leaves or bark:

† A continual spitting.

* The *Quinsy* is a fever attended with difficulty of swallowing, and often of breathing.

568. Or, draw in, as hot as you can bear, (for ten or twelve minutes together) the fumes of *red rose-leaves*, or *camomile-flowers*, boiled in *water* and *vinegar:* or, of a decoction of *bruised hemp-seed*.

This speedily cures the sore-throat, peripneumony, and inflammation of the uvula.——See Extract from Dr. *Tissot*, page 41.

184. *A Quinsy of the Breast*.§

569. Take from eight to twenty drops of *laudanum*, lying down in bed. This helps.

570. Or, make an *issue* in the thigh. This cures.

158. *The Rheumatism*.†

571. To prevent. Wear washed *wool* under the feet.

572. To cure. Use the *cold bath*, with rubbing and sweating:

573. Or, apply *warm steams:*

574. Or, rub in warm *treacle*, and apply to the part brown paper smeared therewith: change it in twelve hours: tried.

575. Or, drink half a pint of *tar-water*, morning and evening:

576. Or, steep six or seven cloves of *garlick*, in half a pint of white wine. Drink it lying down. It sweats, and frequently cures at once.

577. Or, mix flour of *brimstone* with *honey*, in equal quantities. Take three tea-spoonfuls at night, two in the morning; and one afterwards, morning and evening, till cured. This succeeds oftener than any remedy I have found:

578. Or, live on new *milk-whey* and *white-bread* for fourteen days. This has cured in a desperate case.

579. Or, pound the green stalks of *English rhubarb* in *May* or *June*, with an equal quantity of *lump-sugar*. Take the

§ This is known by a sudden unaccountable pain and difficulty of breathing, seizing a person in the night, or on any violent motion.

† Rheumatical pains are generally most violent as soon as you are warm in bed. But there is a cold rheumatism, which is most painful when the part is cold. Constant rubbing will cure this.

quantity of a nutmeg of this three or four times a day. This seldom fails.—See Extract from Dr. *Tissot,* page 61.

In a stubborn rheumatism, let your diet be *barley-gruel,* with *currants, roasted apples, fresh whey,* and *light pudding.*

186. *To restore the Strength after a Rheumatism.*

580. Make a strong broth of *cow-heels,* and wash the parts with it warm twice a day.   It has restored one who was quite a cripple, having no strength left either in his leg, thigh, or loins.

581. Or, mix *gum guaiacum,* (in powder,) with *honey* or *treacle:* take two or three tea-spoonfuls, (or as much as you can bear without purging,) twice or thrice a day. This is the best medicine I have met with for the chronic rheumatism:

582. Or, dissolve one ounce of *gum guaiacum* in three ounces of *spirits of wine.*   Take sixty or eighty drops on loaf-sugar two or three times a day.—This is Dr. HILL's *Essence of Bardana.*

*583. Or, drop thirty drops of *Volatile tincture of guaiacum* on a lump of sugar, and take this in a glass of water every four hours.   It usually cures in a day: tried.

187. *Rickets (to prevent or cure.)*

584. Wash the child every morning in cold water.

188. *Ring-Worms.*†

585. Apply *rotten apples:* or, pounded *garlick:*

586. Or, rub them with the juice of *houseleek:*

587. Or, wash them with *Hungary-water* camphorated:

588. Or, twice a day with oil of *sweet almonds* and oil of *tartar* mixed.

189. *Running at the Nose.*

589. Snuff up a tea-spoonful of Spirits of *hartshorn.*

† Vulgarly called *Tetters.*

98

590. Foment with hot *aqua vitæ* [brandy] for two hours:

591. Or, take *agrimony, spleen-wort, Solomon's seal, straw-berry-roots,* a handful of each; pick and wash them well: stamp, and boil them two hours, in two quarts of white wine in a vessel close stopt. Strain, and drink a large glass of this every morning, and an hour after, drink another. It commonly cures in a fortnight. A good truss mean time is of great use, and perhaps the only thing to be depended on.

592. "I place," says Dr. *Riviere,* "a broad plank sloping from the side of the bed to the ground. On this I lay the patient upon pillows, with his head downward. Then I foment the part for half an hour, with cloths four times doubled, steeped in cold water, gently touching it with my fingers. Afterwards I bind on it, many times doubled, a cloth shaped like a triangle, wet in cold water. ——The gut is generally restored to its place in a few hours. If not, I repeat the operation twice a day, and in two or three days the disease is cured."

191. *A Rupture in Children.*

593. Boil a spoonful of *egg-shells* dried in an oven and pow-dered, in a pint of milk, or three quarters of a pint. Feed the child constantly with bread boiled in this milk.

192. *A windy Rupture.*

594. Warm *cow dung* well; spread it thick on leather, strewing some *cummin seeds* on it, and apply it hot. When cold, put on a new one. It commonly cures a child (keeping his bed) in two days.

193. *A Scald Head.*

595. Anoint it with *Barbadoes tar:*

596. Or, apply daily *white-wine vinegar:* tried.

597. If *wood-soot* is mixed with fresh butter, into an ointment, and the head anointed with it every day, it will generally

cure it at the beginning; but when it is become very bad, a plaister should be made of *gall*, dried to the consistency of a salve, and spread upon linen. This should be applied over the parts affected, and continued on four or five days: then it should be taken off, and the head dressed with the soot-ointment as before.

After the cure, give two or three gentle purges.

If a proper regard was paid to cleanliness in the head and apparel of children, the scald head would seldom be seen.

194. *The Sciatica.**

598. Is certainly cured by a purge taken in a few hours after it begins:

599. Or, use *cold bathing*, and sweat, together with the flesh-brush twice a day:

600. Or, boil *nettles* till soft. Foment with the liquor, then apply the herb as a poultice.——I have known this cure a Sciatica of forty-five years standing:

601. Or, apply *nettles* bruised in a mortar;

602. Or, a mud made of powdered *pitcoal* and warm water. This frequently cures sores, weakness of the limbs, most disorders of the legs, and swellings and stiffness of the joints. It cured a swelling of the elbow-joint, though accompanied with a fistula, arising from a caries of the bone.—See Extract from Dr. *Tissot*, p. 69.

195. *Inflammation or Swelling of the Scrotum.*

603. Wash it thrice a day with strong decoction of *agrimony.*

196. *A Scorbutic Atrophy.†*

604. Use *cold bathing:*——Which also cures all scorbutic pains.

* The *Sciatica* is a violent pain in the hip, chiefly in the joint of the thigh-bone.

† Such a degree of the scurvy as causes the flesh to waste away like a *consumption*.

197. *Scorbutic Gums.*

605. Wash them daily with a decoction of the *Peruvian bark*, adding a little *tincture of roses*, with a solution of *myrrh*.

198. *Scorbutic Sores.*[1]

606. A diet-drink.—Put half a pound of fresh-shaved *lignum guaiacum* (called by the block-makers, *lignum vitæ*,) and half an ounce of *sena* into an earthen pot that holds six quarts. Add five quarts of soft water, and lute the pot close. Set this in a kettle of cold water, and put it over a fire, till it has boiled three hours. Let it stand in the kettle till cold. When it has stood one night, drink daily half a pint, new milk-warm, in the morning, fasting, and at four in the afternoon. Wash with a little of it. In three months all the sores will be dried up: Tried.

199. *The Scurvy.*‡

607. Live on *turnips* for a month:

608. Or, take *tar-water*, morning and evening, for three months:

609. Or, three spoonfuls of *nettle-juice* every morning: tried.

*610. Or, decoction of *Burdock*. Boil three ounces of the dried root in two quarts of water to three pints. Take half a pint daily; unless it purges too much, if so, take less. A decoction of the leaves (boiling one leaf four minutes in a quart of water) has the same effect:

611. Or, take a cupful of the juice of *goose-grass*, in a morning, fasting, for a month: it is frequently called *hariff*,[2] or *cleavers*. Last year I knew many persons cured by it.

‡ The *Scurvy* [Vitamin C deficiency] is known by heaviness of the body, weariness, rottenness of gums, and yellow, lead, or violet-coloured spots on the legs or arms.

N.B. A *Scurvy* attended with *costiveness*, (which is most common,) is termed a *hot-scurvy*; one attended with *looseness*, a *cold-scurvy*.

[1 See *Letters of John Wesley* (Standard Edn), VII. 60.]

[2 Hariff (Etym. doubtful) or Cleavers or Goose Grass—*Galium Aperine*.]

612. Or, pound into a pulp, of *Seville oranges*, sliced, rind and all, and powder-sugar, equal quantities. Take a teaspoonful three or four times a day: tried.

613. Or, squeeze the juice of half a *Seville orange* into a pint of milk over the fire. Sweeten the whey with loaf-sugar, and drink it every morning, new milk warm. To make any whey, milk should be skimmed, after it is boiled.

614. Or, pour three quarts of boiling water, on a quart of *ground malt:* stir them well, and let the mixture stand close covered for four hours: strain it off, and use this as common drink: in hot weather, brew this fresh every day. It will hardly fail.

*615. Or, take morning and evening a spoonful or two of *lemon-juice* and *sugar.* "It is a precious remedy, and well tried."—Dr. *Macbride.*

616. Water and garden cresses, mustard and juice of scurvy-grass help in a cold scurvy.

617. When there is a continual salt taste in the mouth, take a pint of *lime-water* morning and evening.

200. *A broken Shin.*

618. Bind a dry *oak-leaf* upon it:

619. Or, put on a bit of *white paper* moistened with spittle. It will stay on, till the place is well: tried.

This cures a cut also.

201. *Shingles.**

620. Drink *sea-water* every morning for a week, toward the close, bathe also:

621. Or, apply pounded *garlick.*

202. *Sickishness in the Morning.*

622. Eat nothing after six in the evening:

623. Or drink half a pint of water impregnated with *fixed air.*[1]

* A kind of *ring-worm*, which incircles the body, like a belt of a hand's breadth.

[1 See No. 682.]

203. *Sinews shrunk.*

624. Rub the part every morning with *fasting spittle:* tried.

625. Or, beat the yolk of a new-laid *egg*, mix it with a spoonful of water, and rub the part with it before the fire three or four times a day.

204. *Skin rubbed off.*

626. Apply pounded *all-heal.*——It seldom needs repeating.

627. Or, a bit of *white paper* with *spittle.*

205. *Small Pox.*

628. Drink largely of *toast* and *water:*

629. Or, let your whole food be *milk* and *water*, mixed with a little white bread: tried.

630. Or, *milk* and *apples.*

631. Take care to have free, pure and cool air. Therefore open the casement every day: only do not let it chill the patient.

632. If they strike in, and convulsions follow, drink a pint of *cold water* immediately. This instantly stops the convulsions, and drives out the pock: tried.

"There may be pustules a second time, coming out and ripening like the small-pox, but it is barely a cautaneous disorder.

"In violent cases, bleed in the foot; bathe the legs in warm water, twice or thrice a day, before and at the eruption; and apply boiled turnips to the feet. Never keep the head too hot.

"In very low depressed cases, wine may be given: and if the pustules lie buried in the skin, a gentle vomit. In many cases, a gentle purge of *manna,*[1] *cream of tartar,* or *rhubarb.*

"In the Crude Ichorose[2] small-pox, a dish of *coffee* now and then, with a little thick milk in it, has often quieted the vexatious cough.

[1 Manna—An aperient exudation from *Fraxinus ornus.*]
[2 Ichor, a thin, serous fluid from a sore.]

"After the incrustation is formed, change the sick: but let it be with very dry, warm linen." Dr. *Auxham.*

206. *A long running Sore in the Back.*

633. Was entirely cured by eating *betony* in every thing:

634. Or, take every morning two or three spoonfuls of *nettle-juice*, and apply nettles bruised in a mortar to the part. This cures any old sore or ulcer. *I.*

207. *A Sore Leg.*

635. Bind a *diaculum* plaister, an inch broad, round the leg, just above the sore, and foment it, morning and evening, with hot water.

636. Any sore is healed by a plaister of *mutton-suet:* even though it fester or breed *proud flesh.*

208. *A Sore Mouth.*

637. Apply the white of an *egg* beat up with *loaf-sugar:*

638. Or, gargle, with the juice of *cinquefoil:*

639. Or, boil together a pound of *treacle*, three yolks of eggs, an ounce of *bole armoniac*, and the quantity of a *nutmeg* of *alum*, a quarter of an hour. Apply this to the sore part or to an aching tooth: tried.

209. *A Sore Throat.*

640. Take a pint of *cold water* lying down in bed: tried.

641. Or, apply a chin-stay of *roasted figs:*

642. Or, a flannel sprinkled with *spirits of hartshorn* to the throat, rubbing *Hungary-water* on the top of the head: tried.

643. Or, snuff a little *honey* up the nose.

644. An old sore throat was cured by living wholly upon *apples* and *apple water.*

210. *An inflamed Sore Throat.*

645. Lay *nitre* and loaf-sugar mixed on the tongue.

211. *A putrid Sore Throat.*

646. Lay on the tongue a lump of *sugar* dipt in *brandy:* tried.

212. *A Sprain.*

647. Hold the part in very *cold water* for two hours: tried.

648. Or, apply cloths dipt therein, four times doubled, for two hours, changing them as they grow warm:

649. Or, bathe it in good *crab-verjuice:*[1]

650. Or, boil *bran* in *wine vinegar* to a poultice. Apply this warm, and renew it once in twelve hours:

651. Or, mix a little *turpentine* with flour and the yolk of an *egg,* and apply it as a plaister: this cures in a desperate case.

652. Weakness remaining after a sprain, is cured by fomenting the part daily with *beef-brine.*

653. Suppose the ancle sprained. 1. Foment it with warm *vinegar,* four or five minutes every four hours. 2. Stand, if you can, three or four minutes at a time on both your feet, and frequently move the sprained foot. Sometimes also while sitting with your foot on a low stool, move it to and fro. 3. Let it be gently rubbed with a warm hand, at least thrice a day. 4. Two hours after every application of the *vinegar,* let it be just wetted with *spirits of wine,* and then gently rubbed.

213. *A venomous Sting.*

654. Apply the juice of *honey-suckle-leaves:*

655. Or, a poultice of bruised *plantane* and *honey:*

656. Or, take inwardly, one drachm of *black currant-leaves* powdered. It is an excellent counter-poison.

214. *The Sting of a Bee.*

657. Apply *honey.*

[1 An acid liquid expressed from Crab-apples.]

215. *Sting of a Nettle.*

658. Rub the part with juice of *nettles.*

216. *Sting of a Wasp.*

659. Rub the part with the bruised leaves of *houseleek, water-cresses,* or *rue:*

660. Or, apply *treacle,* or *sweet oil:*

661. Or, bruised *onions,* or *garlick.*

217. *Sting of a Bee or Wasp in the Eye.*

662. Apply *carduus* bruised with the white of an *egg:* renew it if it grows dry.

218. *Sting in the Gullet.*

663. Beat well together, with a spoon, some *honey* and *sweet oil* with a little *vinegar;* swallow a spoonful every minute till ease is procured.

219. *A Stitch in the Side.*

664. Apply treacle spread on a hot toast: tried.

220. *Accidental Sickishness, or Pain in the Stomach.*

665. Vomit with a quart of *warm water.* Do this twice or thrice, omitting a day between.

221. *Pain in the Stomach from bad Digestion.*

666. Take fasting, or in the fit, half a pint of *camomile-tea.* Do this five or six mornings:

667. Or, drink the juice of half a large *lemon,* or sweet *orange* immediately after dinner, every day.——Dr. *Mead.*

668. Or, from ten to twenty drops of *Elixir of Vitriol* in *sage-tea,* twice or thrice a day:

669. Or, in the fit, a glass of *vinegar:*

670. Or, take two or three tea-spoonfuls of *Stomachic tincture,* in a glass of water, thrice a day.

☞ The tincture is made thus: *Gentian root* sliced, one ounce: *orange peel* dried half an ounce; *cochineal*, fifteen grains; of *proof-brandy*, one pint: in three or four days it is fit for use.——This is useful in all disorders that arise from a relaxed stomach.

222. *Choleric hot Pains, in the Stomach.*

671. Take half a pint of decoction of *ground-ivy*, with a tea-spoonful of the powder of it, five or six mornings.　*I.*

223. *Coldness of the Stomach.*

672. Take a spoonful of the syrup of the juice of *Carduus Benedictus,*[1] fasting, for three or four mornings.　*I.*

673. Or, chew a leaf of *carduus* every morning, and swallow the spittle; tried.

224. *Pain in the Stomach, with Coldness and Wind.*

674. Swallow five or six corns of *pepper*, for six or seven mornings; tried.

225. *Stone, (to prevent.)*

*675. Eat a small crust of dry bread every morning: tried.

676. Or, drink a pint of *warm water* daily just before dinner. After discharging one stone, this will prevent the generating of another.　Stoop down and raise yourself up again. If you feel pain as if cut through the middle, the pain is not from the *stone*, but *rheumatism*.　Beware of costiveness. Use no violent diuretics.　*Mead* is a proper drink.

677. Or, slice a large *onion;* pour half a pint of *warm water* upon it.　After it has stood twelve hours, drink the water.　Do this every morning till you are well.

[1 *Cnicus Benedictus* or *Blessed Thistle*.]

*678. Beat *onions* into a pulp and apply them as a poultice to the back, or to the groin. It gives speedy ease in the most racking pain: tried.

227. *Stone (to ease or cure.)*

679. Boil half a pound of *parsnips* in a quart of water. Drink a glass of this, morning and evening, and use no other drink all the day.—It usually cures in six weeks:

680. "Or, take morning and evening, a tea-spoonful of *onions*, calcined in a fire-shovel into white ashes, in white wine. An ounce will often dissolve the stone."

681. Or, take a tea-spoonful of *violet seed* powdered morning and evening. It both wastes the stone, and brings it away.

682. Or, drink largely of *water* impregnated with *fixed air*.

Those who have not a convenient apparatus, may substitute the following method:——Dissolve fifteen grains of *salt of tartar* in six spoonfuls of *water*, to which add as much water, acidulated with *oil of vitriol*, as will neutralize the salt. They are to be gradually mixed with each other, so as to prevent the effervescence or dissipation of the fixed air, as much as possible.

228. *Stone in the Kidneys.*

683. Use the *cold bath:*

684. Or, drink half a pint of *water* every morning:

685. Or, boil an ounce of common *thistle-root*, and four drachms of *liquorice* in a pint of water. Drink half of it every morning.

229. *Stoppage in the Kidneys.*

686. Take decoction, or juice, or syrup of *ground-ivy*, morning and evening:

687. Or, half a pint of *tar-water:*

688. Or, twelve grains of *salt of amber* in a little water.

[1 This refers to the extreme pain caused by Stone and not to a fit of madness.]

230. *The Strangury.*[1]

689. Sit over the *steam* of warm water:

690. Or, drink largely of decoction of *turnips*, sweetened with clarified *honey:*

*691. Or, of warm *lemonade:* tried.

692. Or, dissolve half an ounce of *salt-petre* in a quart of water: drink a glass of it every hour.

231. *Sunburn, (smarting.)*

693. Wash the face with *sage-tea.*

232. *A fresh Surfeit.*

694. Take about the size of a nutmeg of the *green* tops of *wormwood.*

233. *To stop profuse sweating.*

695. Drink largely of *cold water.*

234. *To prevent it.*

696. Mix an ounce of tincture of *Peruvian-bark*, with half an ounce of *Spirit of vitriol.*   Take a tea-spoonful morning and night in a glass of water.

235. *To cure Night-Sweats.*

697. Drink a gill of warm *milk*, at lying down.

236. *Swelled Glands in the Neck.*

698. Take *sea-water* every other day.

237. *Indolent Swellings.*

699. Are often cured by *warm steams.*

238. *Soft and flabby Swellings.*

700. Pump *cold water* on them daily:

701. Or, use constant *friction:* or, proper *bandages.*

[1 Strangury—Slow and painful discharge of the Urine, which comes in drops ; cf. ART 271.]

239. *A white Swelling (on the Joints.)*

702. Hold the part half an hour every morning, under a pump or cock. This cures also [all] pains in the joints. It seldom fails: tried.

*703. Or, pour on it daily a stream of *warm water:*

704. Or, a stream of *cold water* one day, and *warm* the next, and so on by turns:

Use these remedies at first, if possible. It is likewise proper to intermix gentle purges, to prevent a relapse:

705. Or, boiled *nettles.*

240. *To dissolve white or hard Swellings.*

706. Take *white roses, elder-flowers, leaves* of *fox-glove*, and of *St. John's wort*, a handful of each: mix with *hog's lard*, and make an ointment:

707. Or, hold them morning and evening in the steam of *vinegar* poured on red hot *flints.*

241. *To fasten the Teeth.*

708. Put powdered *alum* the quantity of a nutmeg, in a quart of *spring-water*, for twenty-four hours. Then strain the water and gargle with it:

709. Or, gargle often with *Phyllerea-leaves* boiled with a little *alum* in *forge-water.*

242. *To clean the Teeth.*

710. Rub them with *ashes* of *burnt bread.*

243. *To prevent the Tooth-Ach.*

711. Wash the mouth with *cold water* every morning, and rinse them after every meal:

712. Or, rub the teeth often with *tobacco-ashes.*

244. *To cure the Tooth-Ach.*

713. Be *electrified* through the teeth: tried.

714. Or, apply to the aching tooth an artificial *magnet:*

715. Or, rub the cheek a quarter of an hour:

716. Or, lay roasted parings of *turnips* as hot as may be behind the ear:

717. Or, put a leaf of *betony*, bruised, up the nose:

*718. Or, lay bruised or boiled *nettles* to the cheek: tried.

*719. Or, lay a clove of *garlick* on the tooth:

720. Or, hold a slice of *apple* lightly boiled between the teeth: tried.

721. Or, keep the feet in warm *water*, and rub them well with bran, just before bed-time: tried.

☞ The first twenty teeth generally last till the sixth or seventh year, they fall out one by one, and are succeeded by others.

The shedding of the teeth is wisely intended, and brought about in a singular manner. Their hardness will not admit of distension like other parts of the body. Hence after an enlargement of the jaw-bone, the original teeth are no longer able to fill up the cavities of it. They must stand unsupported by each other, and leave spaces between them. Under the first teeth therefore is placed a new set, which by constantly pressing upon their roots, rob them of their nourishment, and finally push them out of their sockets.

245. *Tooth-Ach from cold Air*.

722. Keep the mouth full of *warm water*.

246. *Teeth set on Edge*.

723. Rub the tops of the teeth with a dry towel.

☞ There is no such thing as *Worms in the teeth*. Children's using *coral*,[1] is always useless, often hurtful.

[1 A piece of coral hung round the necks of infants for them to bite with their gums whilst teething. "A spoiled child from the time he was in the nurse's arms . . . he threw his coral and bells at my head for refusing him a bit of sugar."—Scott, *The Antiquary*, Ch. 19.]

"*Forcing the teeth into order* is always dangerous.—*Filing* is generally hurtful.

"All rough and cutting *powders* destroy the teeth: so do all common *tinctures*.

"*Sweetmeats* are apt to hurt the teeth, if the mouth be not rinsed after them.—*Cracking nuts* often breaks off the enamel; so does *biting* thread in two.

"Constant use of tooth-picks is a bad practice: constant smoaking of tobacco destroys many good sets of teeth." Mr. *Beardmore*.

247. *Extreme Thirst (without a Fever.)*

724. Drink *spring-water*, in which a little *sal prunellæ* is dissolved.

248. *Pain in the Testicles.*

725. Apply *pellitory of the wall* beaten up into a poultice, changing morning and evening.

249. *Testicles inflamed.*

726. Boil *bean-flour*, in three parts water, one part *vinegar*.

250. *To draw out Thorns, Splinters, and Bones.*

727. Apply *nettle-roots* and *salt:*

728. Or, *turpentine* spread on leather.

251. *Thrush.**

729. Mix juice of *celandine* with *honey* to the thickness of cream. Infuse a little powdered *saffron:* let this simmer awhile and scum it; apply it (where needed) with a feather. At the same time give eight or ten grains of *rhubarb:* to a grown person, twenty.

730. Or, take an ounce of *clarified honey;* having scummed off all the dross from it, put in a drachm of *roche-alum,*

---

* Little white ulcers in the mouth.

finely powdered, and stir them well together. Let the child's mouth be rubbed well with this, five or six times a day, with a bit of rag tied upon the end of a stick: and though it be the thorough thrush, it will cure it in a few days. I never knew it fail.

731. Or, burn *scarlet cloth* to ashes and blow them into the mouth. This seldom fails.

252. *Tonsils swelled.*

732. Wash them with *lavender-water*.

253. *Torpor, (or Numbness of the Limbs.)*

733. Use the *cold-bath*, with rubbing and sweating.

254. *Twisting of the Guts.*

734. Many at the point of death have been cured by taking one, two, or three pounds of *quicksilver*, ounce by ounce. (PAREUS.)

255. *Tympany: or Windy Dropsy.*

735. Use the *cold bath* with purges intermixt:

736. Or, mix the juice of *leeks* and of *elder*. Take two or three spoonfuls of this, morning and evening: tried.

737. Or, eat a few *parched peas* every hour.

256. *A Vein or Sinew cut.*

738. Apply the inner green rind of *hazel* fresh scraped.

257. *The Vertigo: or Swimming in the Head.*

739. Take a *vomit* or two.

740. Or, use the *cold bath* for a month;

741. Or, in a *May* morning, about sun-rise, snuff up daily the dew that is on *mallow-leaves;*

*742. Or, apply to the top of the head, shaven, a plaister of flour of brimstone, and whites of eggs: tried.

743. Or, take every morning, half a drachm of *mustard-seed:*

744. Or, mix together one part of *salt of tartar*, with three parts of *cream of tartar*. Take a tea-spoonful in a glass of water, every morning, fasting. This is serviceable, when the vertigo springs from acid, tough phlegm in the stomach.

258. *Vigilia, Inability to sleep.*

*745. Apply to the forehead for two hours, cloths four times doubled and dipt in *cold water*. I have known this applied to a lying-in woman, and her life saved thereby:

746. Or, take a grain or two of *camphire*. It is both safer and surer than *opium:*

747. *Assa-fætida*, from ten to thirty grains, likewise will in most cases have as much effect as opium.——Drink no green-tea in the afternoon.

259. *Bite of a Viper or Rattle-Snake.*

748. Apply bruised *garlick:*

749. Or, rub the place immediately with *common oil*.—— *Quere*, Would not the same cure the bite of a mad *dog?* Would it not be worth while to make a trial on a *dog?*

260. *To prevent the Bite of a Viper.*

750. Rub the hands with the juice of *radishes*.

261. *An Ulcer.*

751. Dry and powder a *walnut-leaf*, and strew it on, and lay another *walnut-leaf* on that:——Tried.

752. Or, boil *walnut-tree-leaves* in water with a little sugar. Apply a cloth dipt in this, changing it once in two days. This has done wonders:

753. Or, foment morning and evening with a decoction of *walnut-tree-leaves*, and bind the leaves on. This has cured foul bones; yea, and a leprosy; tried.

262. Ulcer in the Bladder or Kidneys.

754. Take decoction of *agrimony* thrice a day:

755. Or, decoction, powder, or syrup of *horse-tail*.

263. Ulcer in the Gum or Jaw.

756. Apply *honey of roses* sharpened with *Spirit of vitriol:*

757. Or, fill the *whites* of eggs boiled hard and slit, with *myrrh* and *sugar-candy* powdered. Tie them up, and hang them on sticks lying across a glass. A liquid distils, with which anoint the sores often in a day.

264. A Fistulous Ulcer.

758. Apply *wood-betony* bruised, changing it daily.

265. A Bleeding Varicuous Ulcer in the Leg.

759. Was cured only by constant *cold bathing*.

266. A Malignant Ulcer.

760. Foment, morning and evening, with a decoction of *mint*. Then sprinkle on it finely powdered *rue:*

761. Or, burn to ashes (but not too long) the gross stalks on which the *red coleworts* grow. Make a plaister with this and fresh butter. Change it once a day:

762. Or, apply a poultice of boiled *parsnips*. This will cure even when the bone is foul:

763. Or, be *electrified:* tried.

267. An Ulcer in the Urethra.†

764. Take a clove of *garlick*, morning and evening.

268. An easy and safe Vomit.

765. Pour a dish of tea on twenty grains of *ipecacuanha*. You may sweeten it if you please. When it has stood four or five minutes, pour the tea clear off, and drink it.

† The *Urethra* is the passage of the urine.

269. *To stop Vomiting.*

*766. Apply a large *onion* slit across the grain, to the pit of the stomach: tried.

767. Or, take a spoonful of *lemon-juice* and six grains of *salt of tartar.*

270. *Bloody Urine.*

768. Take twice a day a pint of decoction of *agrimony:*

769. Or, of decoction of *yarrow.*

271. *Urine by Drops with Heat and Pain.*

770. Drink nothing but *lemonade;* tried.

771. Or, beat up the pulp of five or six roasted *apples* with near a quart of water. Take it at lying down. It commonly cures before morning.

272. *Involuntary Urine.*

772. Use the *cold bath:*

773. Or, take a tea-spoonful of powdered *agrimony* in a little water, morning and evening:

774. Or, a quarter of a pint of *alum-posset-drink*, every night:

775. Or, foment with *rose-leaves* and *plantane-leaves*, boiled in a smith's forge-water. Then apply plaisters of *alum* and *bole armoniac*, made up with *oil* and *vinegar.*

776. Or, apply a *blister* to the Os Sacrum. This seldom fails.

273. *Sharp Urine.*

777. Take two spoonfuls of fresh juice of *ground-ivy.*

274. *Suppression of Urine.*

778. Is sometimes relieved by *bleeding:*

779. Or, drink largely of warm *lemonade:* tried.

780. Or, a scruple of *nitre*, every two hours:

781. Or, take a spoonful of juice of *lemons* sweetened with syrup of *violets:*

782. Or, ten grains of *Mercurias Dulcis.*

275. Uvula† Inflamed.

783. Gargle with a decoction of beaten *hemp-seed:*

784. Or, with a decoction of *dandelion:*

785. Or, touch it frequently with *camphorated spirits of wine.*

276. Uvula relaxed.

786. Bruise the veins of a *cabbage-leaf,* and lay it hot on the crown of the head; repeat, if needed, in two hours.   I never knew it fail:

787. Or, gargle with an infusion of *mustard-seed.*

277. Warts.

788. Rub them daily with a *radish:*

789. Or, with juice of *marigold flowers:* it will hardly fail:

790. Or, water, in which *sal armoniac* is dissolved.

791. Or, apply bruised *purslain* as a poultice, changing it twice a day.   It cures in seven or eight days.

278. Weakness in the Ancles.

792. Hold them in *cold water* a quarter of an hour morning and evening.

279. A soft Wen.

793. Wrap leaves of *sorrel* in a wet paper, and roast them in the embers.   Mix it with finely sifted *ashes* into a poultice.   Apply this warm daily.

794. Dr. *Riviere* says, "I cured a wen as big as a large fist, thus: I made an instrument of hard wood, like the stone with which the painters grind their colours on a marble.

† This is usually called the *Palate of the mouth.*

With this I rubbed it half an hour twice a day. Then I laid on a suppurating plaister very hot, which I kept on four or five days. The wen suppurated and was opened. Afterward all the substance of it turned into matter, and was evacuated. Thus I have cured many since."

280. *The Whites.*

795. Live chastly. Feed sparingly. Use exercise constantly. Sleep moderately, but never lying on your back.

796. Take eight grains of *jalap* every eight days. This usually cures in five weeks:

797. Or, first bleed. Then purge thrice with twenty grains of *rhubarb*, and five of *calomel:*

798. Or, boil four or five leaves of the *white holyhock* in a pint of milk with a little sugar. Then add a tea-spoonful of *Balm of Gilead*. Drink this every morning.—It rarely fails:

799. Or, make *Venice-turpentine, flour*, and *fine sugar*, equal quantities, into small pills. Take three or four of these morning and evening. This also cures most pains in the back:

800. Or, take *yellow rosin*, powdered, one ounce: *conserve of roses*, half an ounce: powdered *rhubarb*, three drachms: syrup, a sufficient quantity to make an electuary. Take a large tea-spoonful of this twice a day, in a cup of *Comfrey-root-tea:*

801. Or, in a quarter of a pint of water, wherein three drachms of *tamarinds*, and a drachm of *Lentisk wood* has been boiled; when cold, infuse *sena*, one drachm, *Coriander-seed* and *liquorice* a drachm and a half each. Let them stand all night. Strain the liquor in the morning, and drink it daily two hours before breakfast:

802. Or, take *quicksilver* and *aqua sulphurata*, as for an asthma.——This seldom fails.

803. Apply *treacle:* tried.

804. Or, *honey* and *flour:* tried.

805. Or, a poultice of *chewed bread.* Shift it once a day:

806. Or, a poultice of powdered *pit-coal*, and warm water.

282. *Worms.**

807. Take two tea-spoonfuls of *brandy* sweetened with loaf-sugar every morning:

808. Or, a spoonful of juice of *lemons:* or, two spoonfuls of *nettle-juice:*

809. Or, boil four ounces of *quicksilver* an hour in a quart of clear water. Pour it off and bottle it up. You may use the same quicksilver again and again. Use this for common drink: or at least night and morning, for a week or two. Then purge off the dead worms with fifteen or twenty grains of *jalap:*

810. Or, take two tea-spoonfuls of *worm-seed*, mixed with *treacle*, for six mornings:

811. Or, one, two or three drachms of powdered *fern-root*, boiled in *mead.* This kills both the flat and round worms. Repeat the medicine from time to time.

812. Or, give one tea-spoonful of syrup of *bear's-foot*[1] at bed-time, and one or two in the morning, for two or three successive days, to children between two and six years of age; regulating the dose according to the strength of the patient.

Syrup of *bear's-foot* is made thus:——Sprinkle the green leaves with vinegar, stamp and strain out the juice, and add to it a sufficient quantity of coarse sugar. This is the most powerful medicine for long round worms.

* A child may be known to have the worms, by chilliness, paleness, hollow eyes, itching of the nose, starting in sleep, and an unusual stinking breath. ——Worms are never found in children that live wholly on milk.

[1 *Helleborus foetidus.*]

Bruising the green leaves of *bear's-foot* and smelling often at them, sometimes expels worms:

813. Or, boil half an ounce of *aloes*, powdered, with a few sprigs of *rue, wormwood* and *camomile*, in half a pint of *gall*, to the consistency of a plaister: spread this on thin leather, and apply it to the stomach, changing it every twelve hours, for three days; then take fifteen grains of *jalap*, and it will bring vast quantities of worms away, some burst, and some alive. This will cure, when no internal medicine avails. See Extract from Dr. *Tissot*, page 145.

283. *Flat Worms*.

814. Mix a table-spoonful of *Norway-tar*, in a pint of *small-beer*. Take it as soon as you can, in the morning, fasting. This brought away a tape-worm thirty-six feet in length:

815. Or, take from two to five grains of *Gamboge*, made into a pill or bolus, in the morning, fasting; drinking after it, a little weak green-tea, and likewise when it begins to operate, till the worm is evacuated. The dose must be regulated according to the patient's strength; for neither this, nor any other medicine, given as an alterative,[1] is of the least service in this disorder. If the head of the worm be fixed in the upper orifice of the stomach, a smart shock from the electrifying-machine will probably dislodge it. Then purge.

To prevent. Avoid drinking stagnated water.

284. Wounds.

If you have not an honest Surgeon at hand.

816. Apply juice or powder of *yarrow: I*.

[1 A medicine which alters. The meaning here is that a mild dose of any medicine just sufficient to alter the course of an illness will have no effect on worms. For an effect on worms it is necessary to give a maximum dose, as much as the patient's strength will tolerate.]

817. Or, bind leaves of *ground-ivy* upon it:

818. Or, *wood-betony* bruised. This quickly heals even cut veins and sinews, and draws out thorns or splinters:

819. Or, keep the part in *cold water* for an hour, keeping the wounds closed with your thumb. Then bind on the thin skin of an *egg-shell* for days or weeks, till it falls off of itself. Regard not, though it prick or shoot for a time.

285. *Inward Wounds.*

820. Infuse *yarrow* twelve hours in warm water. Take a cup of this four times a day.

286. *Putrid Wounds.*

821. Wash them morning and evening with warm decoction of *agrimony*. If they heal too soon, and a matter gathers underneath, apply a poultice of the leaves pounded, changing them once a day till well:

822. Or, apply a *carrot* poultice; but if a gangrene comes on, apply a *wheat-flour* poultice, (after it has been by the fire, till it begins to ferment,) nearly cold. It will not fail.

287. *Wounded Tendons.*

823. Boil *Comfrey-roots* to a thick mucilage or jelly and apply this as a poultice, changing it twice a day.

288. *To open a Wound that is closed too soon.*

824. Apply bruised *centaury*.

Daffy's Elixir.

Take of the best sena, guaiacum, liquorice sliced small, aniseeds, coriander-seeds, and elecampane-root, of each half an ounce: raisins of the sun, stoned, a quarter of a pound; let them all be bruised, and put into a quart of the best brandy. Let it stand by the fire for a few days, then strain it.

Turlington's Balsam.

Take of balsam of Peru, balsam of Tolu, angelica-root, and calamus-root, of each half an ounce: gum storax in tears, and dragon's blood, of each one ounce; gum benjamin, an ounce and a half; hepatic aloes, and frankincense, of each two drachms: let the roots be sliced thin, and the gums bruised; and put all the ingredients into a quart of spirits of wine; set the bottle by the fire in a moderate heat for eight or ten days, then strain it for use.

This is indeed a most excellent medicine, for man, or beast, and for any fresh wound.   I know none like it.

Dr. James's Powders.

Instead of giving half a crown a packet, for these powders, you may at any Druggist's, get Dr. *Hardwick's* fever-powder, for a shilling an ounce, which, (if it be not the same,) will answer just the same end.

COLD-BATHING

Cures Young Children of

CONVULSIONS
Coughs
Cutaneous inflammations, pimples and scabs
Gravel
Inflammations of the ears, navel, and mouth
Rickets
Suppression of urine
Vomiting
Want of sleep

It prevents the Growth of Hereditary

Apoplexies	King's Evil
Asthmas	Melancholy
Blindness	Palsies
Consumptions	Rheumatism
Deafness	Stone
Gout	

It frequently cures every nervous,† and every paralytic disorder: in particular,

The asthma,
Ague of every sort
Atrophy
Blindness*
Cancer
Chin-Cough
Coagulated blood after bruises
Consumptions

† And this, I apprehend, accounts for its frequently curing the bite of a *mad dog*, especially if it be repeated for twenty-five or thirty days successively.

Convulsions
Coughs
Complication of distempers
Conclusive pains*
Deafness*
Dropsy
Epilepsy
Violent fevers
Gout, (running)
Hectic fevers
Hysteric pains*
Incubus
Inflammations*
Involuntary stool or urine*
Lameness
(Old) Leprosy
Lethargy
Loss of appetite, of *smell, *speech, *taste
Nephritic pains
Palpitation of the heart
Pain in the back, joints, *stomach
Rheumatism
Rickets
Rupture
Suffocations
Sciatica
Surfeits (at the beginning)
Scorbutic pains*
Swelling on the joints
Stone in the kidneys
Torpor of the limbs, even when the use of them is lost
Tetanus
Tympany
Vertigo
St. Vitus's dance
Vigilia
Varicous ulcers
The whites.

But in all cases where the nerves are obstructed, (such as are those marked thus*) you should go to bed immediately after, and sweat.

'Tis often necessary to use the *hot bath* a few days before you use the *cold*.

Wise parents should dip their children in cold water every morning, till they are three quarters old: and afterwards their hands and feet.

Washing the head every morning in cold water, prevents rheums, and cures coughs, old head-achs, and sore eyes.

WATER DRINKING generally prevents

Apoplexies, asthmas, convulsions, gout,
Hysteric fits, madness, palsies, stone, trembling.

To this children should be used from their cradles.

The best water to drink, especially for those who are much troubled with the wind, is rain-water. After it has settled, draw it off clear into another vessel, and it will keep sweet for a long time.

ELECTRIFYING, in a proper manner, cures

St. Anthony's fire	Feet violently disordered
Blindness	Felons
Blood extravasated	Fistula Lachrymalis
Bronchocele	Fits
Burns or scalds	Flooding
Coldness in the feet	Ganglions
Contraction of the limbs	Gout
Convulsions	Head-ach
Cramp	Imposthumes
Deafness	Inflammations
Falling sickness	

Involuntary motion of the eye-lids
King's Evil
Knots in the flesh

Lameness
Wasting
Weakness of the legs
Restores bulk and fulness to wasted limbs
Locked jaws and joints
Leprosy
Menstrual obstructions
Ophthalmia
Pain in the stomach
Palsy
Palpitation of the heart
Rheumatism
Ring-worms
Sciatica
Shingles
Sinews shrunk
Spasms
Stiff joints
Sprain, however old
Surfeit
Swellings of all sorts
Sore throat
Tooth-ach
Ulcers
Wens

Drawing sparks removes those tumours on the eye-lids, called barley-corns, by exciting local inflammation, and promoting suppuration.

Nor have I yet known one single instance, wherein it has done harm; so that I cannot but doubt the veracity of those who have affirmed the contrary. Dr. *De Haen* positively affirms, "it can do no hurt in any case:" that is, unless the shock be immoderately strong.

Fasting-spittle outwardly applied every morning, has sometimes relieved and sometimes cured

Blindness
Contracted sinews, from a cut

Corns, (mixt with chewed bread and applied every morning)
Cuts (fresh)
Deafness
Eye-lids, red and inflamed
Scorbutic tetters
Sore legs
Warts

Taken inwardly, it relieves or cures

Asthmas	Leprosy
Cancers	Palsy
Falling sickness	Rheumatism
Gout	Scurvy
Gravel	Stone
King's Evil	Swelled liver

The best way is, to eat about an ounce of hard bread, or sea-biscuit, every morning, fasting two or three hours after. This should be done, in stubborn cases, for a month or six weeks.

₊ I advise all in or near *London*, to buy their Medicines at the Apothecaries' Hall. There they are sure to have them good.

F I N I S.